Juicing for Beginners

The Essential Guide to Juicing Recipes and

Juicing for Weight Loss

Author

Augusta M. Johnson

Contents

PART I:

ALL ABOUT JUICING

Juicing's Advantages

If you're purchasing this book, you're probably already a juicing enthusiast who knows how good it feels to drink freshly squeezed juice. However, if you're searching for reasons to persuade your friends and family to join the juicing revolution, consider the following: • Loss of weight: We are often hungry not because we need more calories, but because our bodies require more nutrients. One glass of juice contains many servings of nutrient-dense fruits and vegetables, and your body absorbs nutrients more easily from juice than from whole food. You may discover that you don't need to eat nearly as frequently or as much when you drink fresh, raw juice.

Healthy Digestive System: There's no denying that digestive

issues are on the increase, particularly in the United States. Everyone I know appears to have a digestive problem at times, whether it's Crohn's disease, ulcers, chronic heartburn, irritable bowel syndrome (IBS), or unexplained nausea, bloating, or stomach aches. While these diseases may be caused by a variety of factors, they all have the same result: it's difficult to obtain the nourishment your body needs to be healthy and whole while you're suffering from one of them. Juicing allows your digestive system to take a break and recover. The juice's vitamins, minerals, and enzymes are rapidly absorbed into your circulation, without straining your digestive systems as the fibres in entire raw vegetables do.

Increased Mental Clarity and Energy: You have more energy for other things, like thinking, when your digestive system has less work to perform. Everyone knows that after a big dinner, you'll probably want to take a lengthy sleep. It takes a lot of energy to digest so much food, so there's not much left over for anything else. A glass of juice is not only easier for your body to digest, but the concentrated nutrients will leave you feeling energised and intellectually alert.

Taste: When it comes to taste, not all vegetable juices are made equal. Perhaps you drank a green drink from a juice stand that made you gag. Healthy juices, on the other hand, may be very tasty! To enhance the taste of any green juice, add some lemon and fresh ginger, or add an apple, pear, or a handful of grapes for added sweetness. Beets and carrots, for example, are naturally sweet veggies that are excellent for encouraging youngsters to enjoy vegetable juices.

Selecting a Juicer

Masticating juicers and centrifugal juicers are the two major kinds of automated juicers (as opposed to manual juicers, which are mostly used for hand squeezing citrus fruits). When you conduct a fast internet search, you'll find that masticating juicers are considerably more costly, beginning at about $200, while a high quality centrifugal juicer can be had for under $100. So, apart from the price, what's the difference?

Centrifugal juicers have an upright design and work by spinning very quickly as the fruit is chewed up, allowing the juice to spin to the container's sides and drain into your cup while the pulp is trapped in the machine's bowl. Centrifugal juicers are simple to operate, fast, and suitable for most fruits and non-leafy vegetables. You can definitely juice leafy greens with a centrifugal juicer (which I do often), but you'll get less juice and more pulp than with a masticating juicer. Wrap your greens around a thick vegetable, like a carrot, to assist them pass down the chute. Wheatgrass also clogs centrifugal juicers, so if you're a huge lover of the grass, you'll want to invest in a masticating juicer or a wheatgrass-specific juicer.

Masticating juicers perform exactly what their name implies: they chew up your produce by crushing and pressing it against the juicer's walls. The juice is then separated from the pulp, providing you with more juice and less pulp than a centrifugal juicer would. Leafy greens juice well with masticating juicers. Large fruit, on the other hand, must be chopped into tiny pieces due to their smaller chutes, which takes a little more time. Some people worry that juicing using a centrifugal juicer warms the produce to the point that some of the enzymes are destroyed, resulting in less nutritional juice. To lose its nutrients, food must be cooked to 118°F, which is unlikely to happen, particularly if you start with cold fruit. However, if you're worried about this, a masticating juicer spins at a considerably slower pace, resulting in less friction and therefore less heating of your fruit.

In a nutshell, here's my juicer recommendation: Get a

centrifugal juicer for about $100–$150 if you want a juicer that works fast and needs little prep time and initial expenditure. Get a masticating juicer in the $200–$300 range if you intend to juice a lot of sprouts and/or wheatgrass, are prepared to spend a few more minutes on prep time, and have the money to put down now (you may wind up saving money in the long run since you'll get more juice from your produce). If money isn't an issue, a masticating juicer in the $500–$600 range can extract even more juice from your fruit while still yielding extremely healthy juice.

Before purchasing a juicer, I suggest doing some research online and reading several juicer reviews. Not all juicers are made equal, but you don't have to spend a lot of money to obtain a decent one.

Produce Selection

The healthiest and most cost-effective method to obtain your juicing components is to grow your own. However, unless you live in a warm area all year, you won't be able to cultivate everything you want to put in your juice all of the time. Consider the following while shopping for produce: 1. Opt for organic. I understand that organic food is generally more costly, and that you can create equally delicious juice from non-organic fruit, but you're presumably juicing for health reasons, and there's no doubt that organic produce is healthier. Even if you properly wash your fruits and veggies, they will have absorbed some of the pesticides and herbicides used on the fields where they were produced, and you don't want to put that material in your body for a variety of reasons. Furthermore, food that is not produced organically has less vitamins and minerals that your body need. If your budget doesn't allow for entirely organic food, go for organic apples, bell peppers, blueberries, celery, cherry tomatoes, collard greens, cucumbers, grapes, hot peppers, kale, lettuce, zucchini, nectarines, and peaches wherever feasible. Pesticide residue is more likely to be found in these areas.

Fresh is the best option. Wilted, slimy, limp, excessively soft, or turning brown fruit should be avoided. Some fruits and vegetables keep for a longer period of time than others. Apples, carrots, and sweet potatoes are examples of dense food that may be purchased in larger quantities since they keep longer. Kale is the green that lasts the longest.

Select a wide range of options. "Everything in proportion," was my grandmother's favourite motto. Your body will not appreciate you if you drink a full head of cabbage every morning. Mix and mix your fruits and vegetables to ensure that you're receiving a diverse variety of nutrients and without overburdening your system.

What You Shouldn't Juice

Some items aren't worth juicing because they're bitter, don't have enough juice to make it worthwhile, or will harm your juicer. Many of these fruits and vegetables are excellent for blending, but juicing would be a waste. You should also only juice fresh fruit—you may mix frozen or thawed produce but not juice it. Also, don't juice any plant parts that you aren't certain are edible. Many different kinds of leaves, stems, and roots should not be eaten. Here's a rundown of some of the most popular items you may believe you can juice but shouldn't: Rinds. Avoid putting rinds through your juicer, with the exception of lemon and lime rinds.

Avocado

Banana\ sCarrot greens (not edible!)

Coconut me

(you can

add
Eggplant

coconut

water to
Green beans

your

juices,
Mustard greens

but

don't

put the Okra

meat

through Onions or leeks

your

juicer)
Papaya peels\sPotatoes (other than sweet potatoes)

(other than sweet potatoes)

Edama

Squashes

Wild parsnips (cultivated ones are fine) (cultivated ones are fine)

A Few Words of Advice

Juicing

isn't rocket science and you shouldn't be intimidated by the process.

But there are a few cautions to keep in mind.

Juicing shouldn't replace eating for long periods of time. Sticking to juice for a few days to detox your body is fine, but juicing removes most of the fibre in your produce, and eventually your body is going to crave that. You can also mix back in some of the pulp to add fibre to your juice.

Not all juices are low calorie. If you're trying to lose weight, avoid or limit produce with the highest sugar content. These include tangerines, cherries, grapes, pomegranates, mangos, figs, and bananas for the fruits. High-sugar veggies include beets, carrots, corn, parsnips, peas, plantains, and sweet potatoes.

It's best to drink your juice right away. It loses

nutrients as it sits, but it will also go bad after a while, even if covered and refrigerated. If you have health issues or are on any medications, it's a good idea to discuss juicing with your doctor. Kale, for example, contains a high concentration of Vitamin K, which promotes blood clotting and can counteract blood thinners. Raw kale can also suppress thyroid function in certain people.

What's the Deal With All That Pulp?

When you see all that pulp piling up in your juicer, you're going to feel wasteful. Unless you use it for something! Here are some ideas: • Compost it!

If you have chickens, they'll eat it.

Mix it into pasta dishes, salads, or into cream cheese or sour cream for a delicious and nutritious dip.

Add it to soups, stews, and broth.

Add it to breads, muffins, cookies, or pancakes. It's not that weird, really. Think about zucchini bread—same idea.

Make crackers!

Tips for a Juicing Detox

A short detox can be a great way to jumpstart weight loss, clear your body of toxins, give your digestive system a break, and get you going on a healthier diet. Here are some tips for your juicing detox.

Plan to detox for 1–3 days. Generally speaking, juice is not meant to replace food for longer than that. Longer detoxes can be helpful in certain situations. If you feel your body needs a 5-or 7-day detox, talk to a doctor and do your own research before you begin.

For 3 days before your detox, start limiting or cutting out completely certain foods and beverages, such as coffee, tea, soda, sugar, meat, dairy, alcohol, and wheat. Easing off these things graduall y make your detox easier and may make it more effective.

During the detox, plan to consume 32 to 96 ounces of juice a day, making sure your juices are at least 50 percent from vegetables.

Drink plenty of water during the detox to clear out your system between juices.

Drink your juices slowly and plan to have one every two hours. This will\shelp to keep your blood sugar even, which helps prevent dizziness, mood swings, and cravings.

If you need to make your juice for the whole day all at once, store the juice you're not going to drink immediately in a glass jar with a tight lid, and keep it refrigerated until you drink it.

Don't plan to be very physically active during your fast. Your body will be processing plenty without the additional strain.

After the detox, reintroduce food gradually over several days.

Healing Chart

If you have a particular condition, use this chart to customise juices to meet your needs.

Condition	Beneficial Juice Ingredients
	Blueberries, Broccoli, Cantaloupe, Carrots, Cherries, Grapes,
Arthritis	
Cancer	

Grapefruits, Kale, Kiwi, Spinach, Strawberries, Papaya, Pineapple, Tangerines, Oranges, Apricots\sApples, Apricots, Beets, Broccoli, Brussels Sprouts, Cabbage, Garlic, Kale, Kiwi, Oranges, Pears, Spinach, Strawberries, Wheatgrass

Diabetes Asparagus, Blueberries, Broccoli, Celery, Cranberries, Raspberries, Spinach, Tomatoes

Digestive Problems

Apples, Blueberries, Cabbage, Carrots, Celery, Mint, Papaya, Parsley, Pineapple Carrots, Ginger, Grapefruits, Lemons, Mint, Oranges, Tangerines

Overweight Apples, Arugula, Broccoli, Brussels Sprouts, Cabbage, Cauliflower, Ginger, Kale, Lemon, Radishes, Turnips, Watercress

Skin Problems

Exhaustion

Apples,

Apricots

, Beets,

Broccoli

,

Cabbag

e,

Carrots,

Cucumb

ers,

Lettuce,

Sprouts,

Sweet

Potatoes

Produce Nutrition Guide

Apples

Apples are full of antioxidants, which boost your immune system and help fight a wide range of diseases. In some studies, apple juice was shown to improve brain function and decrease the risk of Alzheimer's. The phytonutrients in apples also help to regulate your blood sugar. Apple juice has anti- inflammatory and anti-viral properties and helps to detoxify the digestive track.

To juice, cut in halves or quarters and push slowly through the juicer, peels and all. The seeds don't need to be removed as they'll be caught with the pulp.

Beets and Beet Greens

Beet roots (the red part you normally think of when you think of beets) contain calcium, sulphur, iron, potassium, choline, beta-carotene, and Vitamin C. They are also very high in minerals that strengthen the liver and gall bladder and act as the building blocks for blood corpuscles and cells. Just 22 calories of beet greens contain 14 percent of our daily recommended dose of iron, 127 percent of Vitamin A, 50 percent of Vitamin C, and more calcium per calorie than milk. Beets also contain phytochemicals and antioxidants that may help to fight and prevent cancer.

To juice, wash the beet roots well with your hands, removing all dirt, and rinse off the leaves. Juice the roots, stem, and leaves until a stream of brightly coloured juice pours out. When using a centrifugal juicer, alternate between beets and carrots to prevent the beet pulp from building up. When using a masticating juicer, alternate between beets and apples to prevent clogs.

Blueberries\sBlueberries are a good source of colon-cleansing pectin, Vitamin C, K, manganese, and potassium. Plus, blueberries are a fantastic source of antioxidants and anti-inflammatories. Where most fruits have between three and five different kinds of anthocyanin pigments, blueberries have been found to contain as many as twenty-five or thirty. This abundance makes blueberries one of the best foods for protecting our brains as we age, which also means that blueberries may protect from the onset of Alzheimer's disease.

Juicing blueberries is easy. Just rinse them off and pop them into your juicer.

The bouncy little berries have a tendency to try and jump back out again, so make sure to quickly insert your tamper after pouring in the berries. Additionally, try to drink anything made with blueberries within an hour of juicing, as the amount of pectin in blueberries will soon turn any juice made with them into a thick, unappetizing goo.

Broccoli\sBroccoli is a fantastic vegetable that has tonnes of healthy vitamins and minerals. Broccoli is high in Vitamin C, Vitamin A, and also contains iron and calcium. It's also high in protein, Vitamin B1, sulphur, and potassium. Lastly, broccoli is very high in phytochemicals and antioxidants, especially sulforaphane and indoles. Both of these compounds help to cleanse the body of carcinogens and may help to fight cancer.

To juice broccoli, simply wash and cut to fit into the hopper. Alternate with apple to keep everything running smoothly and to reduce strain on your juicer's motor.

Brussels Sprouts

Brussels sprouts may be small, but they're packed with a tonne of nutritious vitamins and minerals. One cup of Brussels sprouts contains only 58 calories, but has 162 percent of your daily recommended dose of Vitamin C and 10 percent of iron. They are also a great source of manganese, potassium, folate, thiamin, riboflavin, and Vitamins B6, A, and K. They also have an impressive amount of phytochemicals, which help to fight cancer.

Juice Brussels sprouts by rinsing them off and dumping them into the juicer.

Carrots

Carrot juice causes the liver to release bile and excess accumulated cholesterol. It also has an alkalizing effect on the blood, soothing the entire nervous system and toning intestinal walls. Carrots help to prevent kidney stones by acting as a detoxifier for the liver and digestive track. Plus, despite one medium carrot having only 30 calories, it contains 330 percent of your daily requirement of Vitamin A. Carrots are also rich in organic calcium, Vitamin C, most of the B vitamins, plus iron, potassium phosphorus, and sodium. The Vitamin A in carrots also acts as an antioxidant that binds to free radicals, which are associated with cancer growth.

To juice your carrots, cut off the tops and the tips and stick them in your juicer. To lighten the flavour of carrot juice, add a half or whole lemon when

juicing.

Celery

Celery juice is a very good source of Vitamin C, folic acid, potassium, and Vitamins B1 and B6. It also has a lot of sodium which, combined with the potassium, make for a great post workout drink. It works to replace electrolytes and offsets muscle cramps and fatigue. In addition to all this, celery juice has a good collection of phytochemicals that helps fight cancer, lower blood pressure, improve the vascular system, and decrease the suffering of migraines.

To juice, simply break off, rinse, and juice the whole stalk, leaves and all. If using a centrifugal juicer, juice the celery last because it is very stringy and can clog the side of the basket.

Cherries

Cherries contain a lot of Vitamin C. They also include quercetin and anthcyanidins, two strong phytochemicals. Both of these things may assist to lower the risk of asthma and lung cancer. Anthcyanidins are just as efficient as aspirin and ibuprofen in reducing inflammation. Finally, cherries are high in melatonin, which is the body's sleep-inducing hormone. Melatonin may assist with sleeplessness as well as depression.

To juice cherries, you must first remove the pits, which may take quite some time.

Cucumbers

Vitamins A, C, and K, as well as phosphorus, pantothenic acid, manganese, magnesium, and potassium, are all abundant in cucumber juice. Cucumbers also contain silicon, a mineral that helps the body's skin, nails, and hair. Silicon also aids in the treatment of insomnia and TB.

Because numerous nutrients are located just under the skin of the cucumber, juice it with the skin on. Cucumbers generate a lot of juice due to their high water content.

Ginger

Ginger is high in Vitamin C, copper, manganese, and potassium, but it is most recognised for its ability to alleviate the symptoms of gastrointestinal problems. It's also well-known as a motion sickness treatment.

illness, particularly for sea sickness, and is, for many individuals, more effective than Dramamine in this respect. Ginger is also an excellent therapy for nausea and vomiting caused by pregnancy because it absorbs gastrointestinal toxins, hormones, and stomach acids. Ginger also includes strong antioxidants called gingerals, which prevent the body from producing inflammatory chemicals and have direct anti-inflammatory actions.

Simply wash the ginger and put it in your juicer, peel and all. Always juice ginger first so that any residual therapeutic volatile oils in the machine may be captured by the other vegetables.

Grapes

Vitamin K, manganese, and potassium are all abundant in grapes. Grapes are well-known for their ability to cleanse the liver and remove uric acid from the body. Flavonoids in red grape juice, particularly from Concord grapes, may inhibit the oxidation of harmful cholesterol, which leads to plaque formation in artery walls. Red grape juice's flavonoids also assist to keep arteries pliable, which helps to avoid atherosclerosis.

Wash the grapes well before placing them in the juicer. You may juice them whole, including the stems. Scrape the peels out of the basket a few times while juicing to prevent the screen from becoming clogged and reducing the output.

Grapefruit

One cup of diced grapefruit provides 120 percent of your daily vitamin C need and 53% of your daily vitamin A requirement. Grapefruit also has a high potassium, thiamin, folate, and magnesium content. Grapefruits also contain a variety of antioxidant-regenerating phytochemicals such as limonene, limonin, nomolin, and naringenin, among others. These phytochemicals may all aid in the prevention of lung and colon cancer.

To juice, use a sharp knife to remove the outer yellow peel away from the white pith as much as possible. Simply put the flesh of the fruit in your juicer after removing the skin. There's no need to strain the seeds out before juicing.

Kale

Kale is unquestionably the king of superfoods. It's high in Vitamin

K, beta-carotene, Vitamin C, lutein, and zeaxanthin, and it's also high in calcium.

Kale provides 200 percent of your daily vitamin C need, 308 percent of your daily vitamin A requirement, and 15% of your daily calcium requirement in only 50 calories. Kale is high in iron, folate, thiamin, riboflavin, magnesium, phosphorus, potassium, copper, and manganese, among other nutrients. Kale is an anti-inflammatory food, a cancer fighter, an anti-depressant in certain instances, and excellent for skin and weight reduction thanks to its minerals.

Kale contains Vitamin K, which helps blood coagulate, so if you're on blood thinners, talk to your doctor before adding it to your drinks. Kale also includes oxalates, which are linked to kidney and gallstone formation. Finally, kale may inhibit thyroid function in certain individuals. Consult your doctor or a naturopath if you have any concerns. It's best to avoid kale juice or consume it just a couple of times a week.

Due to the hardness of its leaves, juicing kale may be difficult. Push the kale through with a slice of apple or a carrot, a bit at a time, during the juicing process to help the procedure go more smoothly.

Lemons

Vitamin C is abundant in lemons. Lemon juice provides 187 percent of your daily Vitamin C requirements and is also an excellent source of folate and potassium. Lemons are excellent for cleansing the body. Lemon juice has a great capacity to breakdown mucus and cleanse toxins from cellular tissue during juice fasts. Lemons are also diuretics and contain the phytochemical limonene, which has been proven to dissolve gallstones and protect against malignancies of all sorts.

Keep part of the white inner peel while juicing lemons to obtain the bioflavonoid limonene. There's no need to strain out the seeds before juicing.

Lettuce

A serving of Romaine lettuce contains 148 percent of the daily required vitamin A, 34 percent of the daily needed vitamin C, and 5% of the daily recommended iron. Vitamin K, thiamin, folate, potassium, manganese, riboflavin, calcium, Vitamin B6, copper, and magnesium are all found in lettuce. Cancer-fighting carotenoids may be found in Romaine lettuce. In addition, the combination of sulphur, chlorine, silicon, and B vitamins promotes good skin and protects against lung cancer.

Simply clean the lettuce leaves and place them in the juicer. Push the button.

a carrot through the foliage

Mint Mint relieves indigestion and inflammation in the stomach, as well as nausea and motion sickness. It may also aid in the relief of nasal, throat, bronchial, and pulmonary congestion. Furthermore, it is a natural stimulant. According to new study, specific enzymes found in mint may help prevent and cure cancer.

Oranges

A single cup of orange juice has 207 percent of your daily Vitamin C requirement. Oranges are high in thiamin, folate, and potassium, among other nutrients. They also include a lot of disease-fighting antioxidants that help the body cleanse itself of free radicals. Orange juice also strengthens your immune system, improves iron absorption, decreases inflammation, lowers blood pressure, and raises good cholesterol while decreasing bad cholesterol.

Cut the skin off oranges with a sharp knife to get the juice. Keep as much of the white pith under the peel as possible, since it's especially high in nutrients.

Parsley

Parsley is a modest herb that is best recognised for its use as a garnish on fine cuisine. But there's a lot more to this unassuming sprig. With just 22 calories, one cup provides 133 percent of our daily required Vitamin C, 101 percent of Vitamin A, and 21% of iron. Fiber, Vitamin K, calcium, magnesium, potassium, copper, and magnesium are all abundant in parsley. Protein, Vitamin E, thiamin, riboflavin, niacin, Vitamin B6, zinc, phosphorus, and pantothenic acid are all excellent sources. Parsley is also a good source of chlorophyll, which works similarly to iron in oxidising the blood. It's also an excellent detox vegetable since it cleanses the kidneys, liver, and urinary system.

It's as simple as washing parsley and putting it in your juicer. Push the parsley through with an apple or a carrot to increase the output.

Pears Pears are high in pectin and fibre, as well as being a rich source of vitamin C.

Copper and potassium, as well as vitamins C, B2, and E. Pears have more pectin than apples, which serves as a diuretic and mild laxative. Pears also contain hydroxycinnamic acid, which helps to prevent stomach cancer and may reduce your chance of getting asthma.

Simply wash the pears and place them in the juicer, skin, stems, and seeds included.

Spinach

Vitamins A, C, and E are abundant in spinach, which was made famous by Popeye. Choline, calcium, potassium, iron, and folic acid are all abundant in this fruit. One cup of spinach juice has 10 grammes of protein, and spinach has 14 times the iron content of red meat per calorie. Spinach is also rich in lutein, an antioxidant that protects your eyes from macular degeneration (an age-related disease that causes blindness) and fights cancer. Glutathione and alpha lipoic acid are abundant in spinach. Glutathione is an antioxidant that protects DNA from oxidation, detoxifies toxins and carcinogens, strengthens the immune system, promotes healthy cellular reproduction, and lowers chronic inflammation. Because alpha lipoic acid is both water and fat soluble, it can protect any cell from oxidative stress.

Most spinach arrives prewashed and may be juiced right away. Simply clean the leaves thoroughly and juice if you have loose spinach or are growing your own.

Strawberries are rich in Vitamin C, with just one cup providing 149 percent of the daily required amount. Strawberries are also high in folate, manganese, potassium, sodium, and iron, among other nutrients. In addition, one-and-a-half cup of strawberries has 3,500 ORAC units, which stands for Oxygen Radical Absorbance Capacity. ORACs are antioxidants that protect us from oxidative damage. Strawberries also protect against free radical damage and contain phenolic acids, which may help to prevent esophageal and colon cancers and promote cancer cell death.

Strawberry juice is simple to make. Rinse them well and juice them whole, stems and all.

PART II:

SMOOTHIES

Green Smoothies: Why, What, How, When, and Where? What are the Benefits of Green Smoothies?

Green smoothies provide a respite from regular meals for your digestive system, resulting in improved energy.

Your consumption of oil and salt is immediately and substantially reduced.

You receive enough greens to feed your body by drinking two to three cups (500–750 ml) of green smoothies daily, and all of the beneficial elements are effectively absorbed.

Your cells are boosted by the chlorophyll, and you shine brighter.

It's a financial investment in your well-being.

You may drop a few additional pounds and go back to your ideal weight.

Your eyes start to twinkle.

Biophotons and living enzymes oxygenate the body and supply

it with calcium, chlorophyll, fluids, and vitality.

What is a Green Smoothie, and how do you make one?

Green leaves, fruit, and water combine to make a healthy drink. The drink's proportions are ideal for humans, with organic, ripe fruit accounting for 60% of the drink and green leaves accounting for 40%.

Victoria Boutenko "created" this cocktail.

It's similar to what chimps consume and "thrive" on. What's the Best Way to Make a Green Smoothie?

What you'll require:

Water, green foliage, and fruit

A knife and a cutting board

For washing your green leaves, use a colander or a salad spinner.

If you want to take your smoothie with you, you'll need a glass, bottle, or thermos.

A mixer, to be precise. Blenders come in a variety of shapes and sizes, as well as a broad range of price and power. It's worth investing in a little more costly blender after you've begun making smoothies. It will be faster and stronger, allowing you to smash frozen fruit and berries, which are used in the tasty green ice cream smoothies.

When Should You Drink Green Smoothies?

Breakfast is the most important meal of the day. It's simple to carry your smoothie to work if you commute by car, bus, or subway.

Snack—instead of coffee, refuel with a smoothie's genuine and simple vitality.

Meal—a fast, easy-to-carry lunch.

The ideal workout meal for before and after your workout. Feel free to amplify.

After a workout, make a smoothie using rice or hemp protein powder.

Dinner—makes the body feel wonderful and allows it to relax overnight. Because the smoothie isn't as taxing on the system as a "normal" supper, you may consume it later in the evening. If you work evenings, it's the ideal time for your body to obtain digestible nutrients and food that moves rapidly through your system.

It's not about drinking a green smoothie at every meal. My buddy began to substitute a smoothie for her breakfast sandwich. She ate normally for the remainder of the day. If you consume five meals each day, you've made a 25% improvement in your total diet. If you wish to cleanse, a green smoothie may be used to replace all of your meals.

What's the Best Place to Get a Green Smoothie?

Green soup is an excellent appetiser or light meal.

At a picnic, that is.

In the company of friends.

You can do this while you're waiting for the metro.

Smoothies may be consumed at any time and in any location!

Smoothies made with greens

Grandma Kale, for example, grows well in the winter and is a wonderful green option.

This is one of my favourite winter greens. 2 cups kale (green)

2 c. liquid

a single apple

a single pear

three occasions

1 tablespoon cuma

In a blender, combine the green kale, water, and minced green kale. Blend in the apple and pear chunks, as well as the pitted dates. Mix with one tablespoon of cuma. More water may be added until the required consistency is achieved.

Smoothie with Asian Greens

Bok choy is a popular Asian vegetable. It's usually steamed or stir-fried, but it's also great in a smoothie as a green foundation!

1 bok choy cup

1 pound of green beans

1 cup sprouted alfalfa

12–1 tablespoon peeled fresh ginger tbsp lime juice 2 cups water two pears

With the water, blend the bok choy, green bean pieces, alfalfa sprouts, and small pieces of peeled ginger. Lime and pear slices should be added. Blend once more. Continually add water until the desired consistency is achieved.

Refresh

Grapefruit has a tart, somewhat bitter flavour that adds to the freshness of the smoothie.

kale (handfuls) 12 cup peeled and segmented water grapefruit

a dozen avocados

Chop the kale and combine it with the water. Blend in the grapefruit segments and the avocado that was scooped out.

Sprout Smoothie

Sprouts contain lots of nutrients and living enzymes, including chlorophyll. Add them to the other greens to optimise your smoothie.

cups spinach

1 cup green lentil sprouts 2 c. liquid

1 large pear\stbsp açaí

½ tbsp of camu camu 1 avocado

Blend spinach and green lentil sprouts with water. Add the chopped pears, açaí, camu camu and mix again. Add the scooped-out avocado. Dilute with water until desired consistency is reached.

Apple Glory

Eating apples every day builds a great foundation for good health. An apple a day keeps the doctor away!

apples

2 cups spinach

2 c. liquid

a dozen avocados

Chop the apple into pieces and blend it with spinach and water. Mix again.

Continually add water until the desired consistency is achieved.

Cacao Dessert Smoothie

A smoothie that's lunch and dessert in one! 2 handfuls of kale

2 cups of water 2 dates

2 tbsps raw cacao powder 1 tbsp honey

avocado

Chop the kale and mix with the water. Add the pitted dates, cacao, and honey and blend again. Add scooped-out avocado and more water until desired consistency is reached.

Green Pear Smoothie

Use ripe pears for a smoother and creamier smoothie. 2 large handfuls of kale\scups water

2 large pears, ripe\scup blueberries, frozen

Blend chopped kale with the water. Add pieces of pears and

blueberries and mix again. Dilute with water for desired consistency.

Daily Green Smoothie

Many of the green smoothies are based on what you have at home. Here is a variation on my "I'll use what I have" smoothie!

cups mixed salad 2 c. liquid

½ cup broccoli

½ inch cucumber 1 kiwi

two pears

a dozen avocados

Mix the salad with the water. Add pieces of broccoli and cucumber.

Blend. Add pieces of kiwi and pears. Scoop out the avocado and mix into the smoothie. More water may be added until the required consistency is achieved.

Garden Smoothie

Wild leaves are really the best green leaves that you can use in your smoothie. Miner's lettuce is one of my favourites, and it grows right outside my house. Organic, locally grown, and free!

2 cups miner's lettuce (or other wild green leaves) (or other wild green leaves) 1 tbsp hemp protein powder

1–2 cups water

2 cups honeydew melon

Mix miner's lettuce with hemp seed protein powder and water. Cut honeydew melon into pieces and add to mixture. More water may be added until the required consistency is achieved.

Fresh!

Serve with ice cubes for a really fresh and delicious smoothie. Mint is also good for digestion.

cup mint

1–2 cups water

pears\stbsp lime juice

Blend chopped mint with one cup of water. Add cut-up pears and lime juice, and mix again. Dilute with more water until desired consistency is reached.

Strawberrylicious

Fresh and cool strawberry smoothie! Basil and strawberries are both rich in iron.

cups strawberries

2 cups basil

1 tbsp lime juice

1 cup water

½ cup ice cubes

Optional; honey to sweeten

Mix strawberries, basil, lime juice, and water. Add ice cubes and mix again. Green Lúcuma Smoothie

Lúcuma is a superfood that contains high levels of B3 and iron and gives the smoothie a creamy, caramel flavour.

1½ cups lettuce 2 c. liquid

a single pear

1 apple\ssmall zucchini\stbsps lúcuma

Chop the lettuce and mix with water. Cut the pear, apple, and zucchini into pieces and add. Blend once more. Add the lúcuma and dilute with water until desired consistency is reached.

Green Smoothie with Chaga Tea

Chaga grows on trees and is super-nutritious and especially rich in antioxidants. It's the perfect base for a green smoothie.

2 cups spinach 2 cups chaga tea 2 celery stalks

½ cucumber a single apple

⅛ inch ginger, peeled 1 avocado

Blend spinach with chaga tea. Cut celery, cucumber, ginger, and apple into pieces. Add the ingredients to the blender and mix. Scoop out the avocado and add more water until desired consistency is reached.

Sea-buckthorn Smoothie

Sea-buckthorn can be purchased fresh or frozen. It's rich in

Vitamin C and antioxidants, which make your skin glow.

1 cup lettuce\scup sunflower shoots 1 cup sea-buckthorn\scups water

Mix all the ingredients with water. More water may be added until the required consistency is achieved.

Green Orange

Spruce up your traditional orange juice with spinach. Kids love it! 2 cups orange juice

2 cups spinach

Blend the ingredients and enjoy!

Iron Smoothie

Parsley contains lots of iron, which is especially good for women. 2 cups flat-leaf parsley

2 c. liquid

2 apples

1 zucchini

1 tbsp lemon juice

Mix parsley with water. Cut apples and zucchini into pieces. Add remaining ingredients and blend again. Dilute with more water until desired consistency is reached.

Green Kiwi Smoothie

Kiwi is a fruit that isn't too sweet and gives the smoothie a tart, fresh taste reminiscent of yoghurt.

6 inch cucumber

kiwi\scups lettuce

1 tbsp lemon juice 1 avocado\stbsp lemon juice 1–2 cups of water

Cut the cucumber and kiwi into chunks. Mix together with lettuce, scooped- out avocado, lemon juice, and water. Dilute with water until desired consistency is reached.

Apricot & Melon Smoothie

This is a real summer smoothie with melon and fresh orange apricots. It's spiked with the power of sunflower shoots and spinach, and it's also hydrating because of the cucumber and water. Bring it in a thermos to the beach!

cups melon

4 inches cucumber

1 cup apricot

1 cup spinach

1 cup sunflower shoots 2 c. liquid

Cut the melon, cucumber, and apricots into chunks. Mix with spinach, sunflower shoots, and water. Dilute with water until desired consistency is reached.

Green Passion\sPassion fruit gives this smoothie a tart flavour, and the creaminess derives from the banana . . . Exotic!

cup spinach\scups water

passion fruits

2 bananas

Blend the spinach with water. Scoop out the pulp from the passion fruit and add together with peeled and sliced bananas. Mix. More water may be added until the required consistency is achieved.

Green Broccoli Smoothie

Broccoli contains more starch than green leaves, which makes for a more filling smoothie!

cup broccoli\spears

1 cup spinach

1 cup sunflower shoots 3 tbsps lemon juice

3 cups water

Cut the broccoli and pear into pieces. Mix with spinach, sunflower shoots, lemon juice and water. Dilute with more water until desired consistency is reached.

Apple Green

Arugula has a spicy taste and adds a peppery flavour to the smoothie. The bitterness of the arugula promotes digestion.

2 handfuls of arugula 1–2 cups water

2 apples, red\s½ inch cucumber 1 tsp lemon juice

a dozen avocados

Blend arugula with 1 cup of water. Cut the apple and cucumber into pieces. Add the remaining ingredients, except for the avocado, and blend again. Add the scooped-out avocado and mix, dilute with water until desired consistency is reached.

Pomegreen Smoothie

Tip! To pick out the small red pomegranate seeds, cut the fruit in half, gently squeeze the skin, and turn it inside out over a bowl. Remove the seeds. Discard the white parts of the skin, which can taste bitter. Strain the juice, pour into a beautiful glass, and add the kernels to the smoothie.

2 cups salad

1–2 cups water

2 pears\scup (about ½ pomegranate) pomegranate kernels

Blend the salad with 1 cup of

water. Cut the pear into pieces and add the other ingredients before mixing again. More water may be added until the required consistency is achieved.

Green Grape Smoothie

Whenever you buy grapes, you should look for organic ones with seeds. 2 cups crisp lettuce\scups water

2 cups green grapes with seeds a single pear

Blend the crispy salad with water. Seed grapes and cut the pear into pieces. Add the remaining ingredients and

blend again. Dilute with more

water until desired

consistency is reached.

Apple Pie Smoothie

With a little imagination, this

smoothie resembles a

scrumptious apple pie! 2

handfuls of spinach

1–2 cups water

2 red apples

2 tbsp lúcuma powder 1–2

tsps cinnamon

Blend the spinach with 1 cup

of water. Cut the apple into

pieces. Add the remaining

ingredients and mix again.

Dilute with water until desired

consistency is reached.

Green Christmas Smoothie

Sharon is a typical Christmas

fruit. Don't worry if the fruit

has some brown spots, as it's

just a little sugar that has

precipitated in the skin.

2 handfuls of kale 2–3 cups of

water

large persimmon or two

sharon fruit 1–2 tsps

cinnamon

Chop kale and mix with 1 cup

of water. Cut

persimmons/sharon into

pieces and add together with cinnamon. Mix again. Continually add water until the desired consistency is achieved.

Papaya with Lime Smoothie

Papaya contains an extremely beneficial enzyme that helps our digestive system.

handfuls of spinach 1–2 cups water

¼ large papaya

½ lime juice

Blend the spinach and 1 cup of water. Add chunks of papaya and lime juice and mix again. Continually add water until the desired consistency is achieved.

Ginger Green Smoothie 2 handfuls of kale

2 c. liquid

6 soaked figs, soaked 2–4 hours

½ inch ginger

Chop the kale and mix with 1 cup of water. Add figs and peeled, chopped ginger and blend again. Continually add water until the desired consistency is achieved.

Green Creamy Apricot

Smoothie

Dried apricots should be brown. Avoid buying the orange ones, which are sulfurized, meaning that sulphur has been added. This is done to inhibit bacteria and fungi and to preserve the colour. However, this can also cause asthma.

1 cup nettle

1 cup spinach

½ cup of soaking water 1½ cup water

1 red apple

8 soaked apricots, soaked 2–4 hours

Chop the nettles and mix with spinach, water, and the water from the apricots. Add pieces of apples and apricots, and mix again.

Col. Mustard Greens

2 cups mustard greens 2–3 roma tomatoes ¼ avocado

1 small zucchini

1 lime

Favorite herbs to taste

Blend with water to desired consistency.

Works well with fresh oregano, basil, or dill, but feel

free to experiment with other

fresh herbs.

What-A-Lemon

2–4 cups watermelon

1 bunch watercress

1 roma tomato ½ lemon

1 tbsp olive oil

Blend with ice to desired

consistency.

Apple Sprouts

¼ of a small red onion a

single apple

a single pear

1 handful spinach

3–4 Brussels sprouts

Ginger to taste

Blend with ice to desired

consistency.

Sangria Blanca

1–2 white peaches (pitted) 1

cup rainier cherries (pitted) 1–

2 white nectarines (pitted) 1

cup green grapes

6–10 endive leaves

3–5 mint leaves

Blend with ice to desired

consistency.

Mangomole 1 mango

1 peach

1 handful spinach

1 small bunch cilantro ¼

small onion ¼ avocado

½ yellow bell pepper Jalapeño

to taste

½ lemon (peeled)

Blend with ice to desired

consistency.

Gazpacho

1–2 roma tomatoes

½ red bell pepper 1 garlic

clove ¼ small onion

1 handful cilantro

1 handful parsley Jalapeño to

taste

Tarragon to taste

Blend with ice to desired

consistency.

Cosmo Chiller

1–2 cups mustard greens 1

medium cucumber

1 cup frozen cranberries 1

lime (peeled) ½ lemon

(peeled) 3–5 mint leaves

Blend with ice to desired

consistency.

Blue Banana Green Smoothie

1 frozen banana (ripe)

A handful of blueberries 2

inches of cucumber 1–2

cups of almond milk

baby spinach, a

handful 1 tsp honey

or less

Optional Ice Extras:

Watercress, a

handful

Simply combine all

ingredients in a

blender and mix on

low until smooth.

Blend with a few ice

cubes and increase

the speed.

If you use almonds

and water instead of

almond milk, your smoothie will be crunchier.

Smoothie with Cacao and Greens

1 banana, frozen

a half apple

1 tsp cacao powder

(organic) a couple of

handfuls of baby

spinach 1 tsp flax

seed, heaping a cup

or two of water

Optional Add-Ons:

1 teaspoon cacao

nibs (will be a little
crunchy)

a splash of vanilla
extract or a few
scrapes of a vanilla
pod (sugar-free)

Combine all
ingredients in a
blender. This
smoothie may be a
bit thin for your
tastes, so add some
ice and mix to
thicken it up without
adding any
additional
ingredients. If you

don't have any,

throw in an avocado.

Green Smoothie with

Berries and Melon 1

cup raspberry berries

a few cantaloupe

melon pieces 1

banana and a handful

of fresh spring

greens a cup or two

of water

Optional Add-Ons:

a bunch of broccoli

or alfalfa seeds that

have sprouted

To smooth out the

spinach leaves,

combine all of the

ingredients in a

blender and mix on

low for a few

seconds before

increasing to high.

Green Smoothie with

Pineapple Detox

a little amount of

ginger grated 1

pound pineapple

1 avocado 1

cucumber inch

Several Romaine

lettuce leaves Water

(about 2 cups)

Optional Add-Ons:

For even more

detoxifying, add

some celery.

To begin, combine

the cucumber and

pineapple in a

blender with a little

water. Then add the

other ingredients to

the blender and mix

until smooth.

Smoothie with a kick

of spring greens

12 lemons squeezed

handfuls of kale or

spinach a single

apple

1 banana, frozen

a single avocado

chia seeds, 1 tbsp

Water (about 1–2

cups) 1 quart ice

Blend all ingredients

till smooth, except

the ice, then add the

ice and smooth it up.

Smoothie with

Berry, Rocket, and

Greens

1 banana, frozen

strawberries, 1 cup

blackberries, 1 cup

arugula or rocket

lettuce, a bunch

coconut milk (about

2 cups)

Blend all of the

ingredients together

until smooth. Green

Smoothie with Pears

pears

a single avocado

1 tblsp. lamb's

lettuce

1 handful cilantro or

coriander Water

(about 2 cups)

1 tblsp maca

(optional)

If you need a bit

more sweetness, add

a little honey.

Combine all

ingredients in a

blender with ice until

smooth. Taste, and if

your pears aren't

very sweet, drizzle

with honey.

Green Smoothie in a

Hurry

spinach, 1 handful

1 frozen banana 1

tiny pinch of parsley

1 papaya (fruit)

(seeds removed)

a few cubes of ice a

cup or two of water

In a blender,

combine all

ingredients and mix

until smooth. If you

aren't accustomed to

the flavour of

parsley, add extra

banana or prepare it

with only a sprig or

two.

Green Smoothie with

Orange for Breakfast

2 swiss chard or
lettuce leaves, big 1
orange (whole,
without seeds or
peel)

12 grapefruit
(seedless and
peelless) a single
avocado

a single banana

Cubes of ice

a cup or two of water

Optional Add-Ons:

1 tbsp vanilla rice
protein powder and a

sprinkling of oats

Combine all

ingredients in a

blender and mix until

smooth—then dash

out the door!

Smoothie with

Orange and Go

Green

a single orange

a single avocado

spinach, 1 handful

a cup or two of

almond milk

Optional Add-Ons:

Some cucumbers and

lettuce Combine all
of the ingredients in
a blender and get
ready to go!

Green Smoothie with
Choco Passion
handfuls of frozen
bananas spinach
passion fruit (the
insides)
1 tsp cocoa powder
or dark chocolate
chunks 2 cups
almond milk (about)
In a blender,
combine all of the

ingredients.

Smoothie with Sweet

Greens

kale, 2 handfuls 1

banana pear

a handful or two of

dates 1 cup of liquid

Ice

Combine everything

in a blender. To

make it even

sweeter, add a

teaspoon of honey.

Melon & Strawberry

Green Smoothie with

a Twist

swiss chard (cups)

watermelon, 2 cups

cucumber, 2 inches a

single avocado

1 tblsp. chia seeds

1 lemon squeezed a

cup or two of water

Ice

With the exception

of the ice, combine

all ingredients in a

mixing bowl. Blend

till smooth, then add

the ice to chill it

down.

Smoothie with

Tropical Greens 1

pineapple chunks

cup 1 mango (cup)

spinach, 1 handful

12 cup coconut milk,

coconut water, or a

little amount of

coconut cream

a glass of water

a little amount of ice

In a blender,

combine all of the

ingredients and mix

until smooth. At the

very end, add ice.

Taste and adjust the amount of coconut or water according on your preferences.

Green Smoothie to Wake You Up

1 celery stalk 1 cup spinach

A chunk of

cucumber 1 frozen

banana

1 cup of raspberries

½–1 avocado

1 cup of cantaloupe melon

chunks 1–2 cups of water

Combine all ingredients and mix until

smooth. Fruity Power Green

Smoothie

2 cups of swiss chard or

kale A few arugula

(rocket) leaves 1 kiwi

1 banana

1 peach (pitted)

1 tsp of

wheatgrass 1–2

cups of water

Blend all ingredients together until

smooth. Breakfast Filler Green

Smoothie

1 apple

½–1 avocado

1 cup of

blueberries 2

handfuls of

spinach

1 tsp of chocolate powder or a tbsp of

cacao nibs 1 tbsp of instant oats (or pre-

blended oats)

1 cup of water or green or white tea (chilled)

a few ice cubes

Blend all of the ingredients together, then smash the ice.

Green Smoothie Booster for Lunch

1 big pineapple slice 3 romaine lettuce leaves

a dozen avocados

1 handful leaves of spinach 1 banana, frozen

tbsp flax seed or chia seed milled glasses of water 1 teaspoon

maca root

Combine all ingredients in a blender and blend until smooth.

For a thicker, sweeter smoothie, add additional banana.

Smoothies with Protein

Punch made with peaches peaches (two)

a single mango

1 lettuce bunch (red leaf or mixed)

Remove the mango peel as well as all of the pits (stones).

Blend with ice or water. Whey protein powder is an optional protein source.

Plumkin

1–2 tblsp. pumpkin purée plums, 1–2 (pitted)

1 big handful spinach, seasoned to taste with cinnamon 2 quarts coconut milk

Blend until smooth, adding additional coconut water if needed.

To create the ideal post-workout recovery green smoothie, include whole milk, chia seeds, or your favourite protein powder.

Plain whole milk yoghurt is an optional source of protein.

Simply Sweet

2–4 leaves of kale (de-stemmed) strawberries, 1–2 cups

a single banana

To get the required consistency, add water and ice to the

blender. Whey protein powder is an optional protein source.

Minty Sweet

1–2 collard leaves, big 1 kiwi 1 pear (peeled)

1 pound of blackberries

1 pound of blueberries

3–6 leaves of mint

To get the required consistency, add water and ice to the

blender. Chia seeds are an optional source of protein.

1 cup pineapple orange (peeled) leaves rainbow chard Pia

Kale-ada

2 leaves of kale (stemmed) a single banana

1 quart of coconut milk

Blend with ice until desired consistency is achieved. Whey protein powder is an optional protein source.

Honey from the wild

3–4 kale leaves, big (stemmed) 2–4 big basil leaves

1 pound of blackberries

a single banana

1 tablespoon honey

To get the required consistency, add water and ice to the blender. Optional protein sources: Plain yoghurt made with whole milk

Candy made with chard

chard leaves, 2–4 a cup or two of red grapes 2–3 occasions

(pitted)

1 tablespoon of almond butter

To get the required consistency, add water and ice to the blender. Optional protein sources: Whole, unpasteurized milk

Mocha Cocoa

2–3 leaves of kale (stemmed) 1 bunch of mixed greens

a single apple

1 tbsp almond butter 1 banana

1–2 tbsp cocoa powder (raw) to taste vanilla To get the required consistency, add water and ice to the blender. Instead of using vanilla extract, try finding some vanilla beans and cutting them open, scraping out the insides, and using that instead. They're tasty, and you get rid of the alcohol in extracts, however little it may be.

Egg protein powder is an optional protein.

Smoothies made with yoghurt Cups of honeydew melon, sliced into pieces Apple & Melon Smoothie a single apple

2 tbsp live organic yoghurt (greek yoghurt is nice and thick)

lime juice, 1 tbsp

1 cup of liquid

Cubes of ice

Blend all of the ingredients together until smooth. Smoothie with Coco and Mango

1 mango banana pineapple slices juiced 1 tbsp coconut cream,

1 cup coconut milk, or 1 cup of water

Water

Ice

Simply combine the ingredients in a blender and mix until smooth. It's ideal for a fast burst of fruit.

Smoothie with Melon and Berry Yogurt

12 melon cantaloupe strawberries, 1 cup

a dozen bananas

1 cup of living food (healthy bacteria included) yoghurt In a blender, combine all of the ingredients.

Diet Yogurt Smoothie with Grapefruit and Pineapple

Several pineapple slices 1 avocado, tiny

a few lettuce leaves

a grapefruit (12 oz.)

a generous pinch of lime

1 cup live low-fat yoghurt

If required, add more water to thin it out. Combine all ingredients in a blender and blend until smooth.

Strawberries & Pomegranate Smoothie

12 cup freshly squeezed pomegranate juice a single banana strawberries, a handful (or mixed frozen berries) 1 big tablespoon crème fraîche or regular low-fat yoghurt 1 tblsp honey (optional)

1 cup of liquid

Ice

In a blender, combine all of the ingredients and mix until smooth. Smoothie with Sweet Yogurt and Watermelon

a cup of naturally fermented Greek yoghurt cups of watermelon 1 tbsp honey

a dozen cucumbers (optional) two occasions (optional)

If required, add more water.

To make a thick smoothie, combine all of the ingredients in a blender. Apple Cinnamon Smoothie

2 pears

a single banana

1–2 tablespoons greek yoghurt with probiotics cinnamon (1 tsp)

1 tblsp honey

1 cup almond milk (about) (or water and a handful of

almonds for a thicker smoothie)

Ice

Combine all ingredients in a blender and blend until smooth.

Check consistency by adding a few cubes of ice as you go.

PART III:

JUICES

Fruit Juices The Quick and Dirty Flu Fighter 2 small–medium oranges, peeled 1 small grapefruit, peeled\s½ lemon

1 Yellow or McIntosh apple (or any other sweet apple) (or any other sweet apple)

A small chunk of ginger Optional Additions:

A handful of parsley Replacements:

1 cup peeled pineapple for apple The Tart and Sweet Cooler cup cranberries

½ cup raspberries\scups pineapple, peeled Optional Additions:

½ lemon Replacements:\sUse either cranberries or raspberries if you have only one.

The Lola Dreaming

4 small Persian cucumbers 2 cups of baby spinach

A handful of mint

1 small yellow delicious apple 6–8 strawberries

lime kiwis

Optional Additions:

A small chunk of ginger Replacements:

Lemon for lime

Pear for apple

The Berry Melon Heaven 10–12 strawberries

½–⅔ of a medium cantaloupe, peeled Optional Additions:

A few chunks of pineapple Replacements:

Honeydew for cantaloupe The Sweet Pear Sensation 2 small pears, any kind

1 medium sweet apple 2–4 stalks celery ½ lemon

A small chunk of ginger Optional Additions:

3–4 strawberries or 4–5 raspberries Replacements:

Pineapple for apple

The Wake Me Up Morning Cocktail 2 cups fresh cranberries

2–3 medium carrots

A handful of cilantro 2 oranges, peeled apple

Optional Additions:

2–4 strawberries or raspberries Replacements:

Parsley or dill for cilantro

All oranges or all apples The Pomegranate Pow Wow 1 large pomegranate, peeled ½–1 lime medium sweet apples, any kind Optional

Additions:

None Replacements:

Lemon for lime

The Sunrise in Paradise 2 mangoes, peeled

2 sweet delicious apples Optional Additions: 2–4 strawberries

Ginger to taste Replacements:

Pear for apple The Pink Silk ⅓ or ½ medium watermelon, peeled

Optional Additions:

A handful of fresh mint

½ lime Replacements:

Basil or dill for mint leaves

The Orange Ecstasy 3–4 medium carrots 2 oranges, peeled

A small chunk of ginger Optional Additions:

½ lemon Antioxidant Rush 1 cup blueberries cup cherries apples

Blueberries, cherries, and apples are all chock-full of antioxidants. All three are also anti-inflammatories, which can help with a wide range of conditions, including arthritis, chronic pain, heart disease, and even depression.

The Ruby Rapture 4 blood red oranges 8–10 strawberries Pear Delight

2 pears

2 cucumbers

½ lemon

½ cup strawberries or raspberries

The pectin in pears is a type of fibre that is not lost when the fruit is juiced, making it good for colonic health. Pears also contain antioxidants that protect against brain aging. Berries are also full of antioxidants.

Tropical Punch

2 mangoes, peeled

1 cup pineapple cup berries, any kind

Mangoes are a good source of Vitamin C, Vitamin A, and quercetin, which helps to protect against cancer. Pineapple contains lots of Vitamin C and the enzyme bromelain, which reduces inflammation and supports digestive function. Berries are full of antioxidants.

Melon Refresher

¼ medium watermelon, flesh only ½ cantaloupe, flesh only 1 cup mint leaves

Watermelon contains Vitamins A, B1, B6, and C. Its high water content makes it incredibly hydrating and refreshing. Cantaloupe is high in Vitamins A and C and contains Vitamins B1, B6, and potassium.

They help reduce anxiety and depression, and help fight intestinal and skin cancer, as well as cataracts. Mint leaves freshen breath and soothe the stomach.

Very Berry cups strawberries

2 cups blueberries

2 cups raspberries or blackberries

Blueberries and blackberries contain anthocyanins, antioxidants that protect artery walls from damage caused by free radicals. Blackberries are also beneficial for skin. Strawberries are full of Vitamin C and antioxidants that protect the brain.

Juices from Vegetables

The Ultimate Purifier 2 Persian

cucumbers 1 medium beet 14 cabbage

head

1 parsnip, medium

a bunch of parsley a big delicious apple,

yellow or red a single lime

Additions that are optional:

To make it less sweet, add a handful of

beet top greens (2–3).

Replacements: ginger and garlic to taste

For lime, use lemon.

Carrots as a substitute for parsnips

The Lagoon with Crystal Clear Water

Cucumber, big

a few sprigs of parsley celery stems, 3–4

3–4 carrots, medium 14 fennel bulb and

1 tiny delicious pear stem 1 Belgian

endive (whole) Additions that are

optional:

Watercress, a tiny handful

Turmeric, a tiny piece 1–2 garlic cloves,

peeled Replacements:

For Belgian endive, more carrots

Pear for apple

Any other cucumbers available? Multi-

Nutrient Juice 6 Swiss chard leaves

a beet, a beet, a beet, a beet

3–4 carrots, medium

4 tomatoes (roma)

parsley, a handful 1–2 cucumbers, tiny

a single lemon

a ginger root piece Additions that are

optional:

1–2 garlic cloves, peeled

To make it less sweet, add a handful of

beet top greens (2–3). Replacements:

Cucumbers with celery

Swiss chard may be substituted with kale.

The Winter Healer in Its Entirety 4–5 Swiss chard leaves 3–4 lettuce leaves

2–3 carrots, medium

medium sized beet

2–3 cucumbers, tiny

Watercress with Roma tomatoes in a bunch

12 lemon or lime cloves garlic cloves, peeled

a ginger root piece Additions that are optional:

To make it less sweet, add a handful of beet top greens (2–3). To make it less sweet, add a handful of carrot top greens (2–3). Replacements:

Watercress with parsley

Swiss chard with spinach

Pallooza

XXXXXXXXXXXXXXXXXXXX 4 celery stalks 1 cup spinach

3–4 broccoli stalks and florets

12 bunch parsley Granny Smith green apples, tiny 2 garlic cloves

1 tiny ginger chunk

1 seedless jalapeo pepper Additions that are optional:

1 tiny turmeric chunk Replacements:

Cilantro in place of parsley

Apples for carrots

Super Detoxes aplenty 6–8 kale leaves

4–6 celery stalks entire Belgian endive

12 onion, white

red delicious apples, tiny

12 lime or lemon 1 ginger chunk

two garlic cloves 1 teaspoon cayenne

pepper

Additions that are optional:

watercress, a tiny handful

Replacements:

Kale with collard greens

Belgian endive with cabbage

Heavenly Concoction of Red and Green

3–4 carrots, medium

6–8 kale leaves

13 fennel bulb and stem

12 bunch dill or mint 3–4 tomatoes,

Roma 3–4 broccoli florets

12 big cucumbers (Italian) a single

lemon

Additions that are optional:

a dozen bunches of watercress

1–2 garlic cloves, peeled Replacements:

Kale may be substituted with spinach.

For cilantro, use dill.

The Green Juice of Mamma 2 tomatoes,

Roma

2–3 carrots, medium

parsnips, small

1 cucumber from Italy 1 cup spinach,

baby

1 tablespoon cilantro 1 handful of

parsley

14 fennel sprigs

1 cayenne pepper, tiny (or spice powder

to taste) Additions that are optional:

to taste garlic and ginger Replacements:

More parsley for cilantro, or the other

way around Cayenne pepper may be

replaced with jalapeo pepper.

Carrots, carrots, carrots, carrots, carrots, carrots, carrots, carrot The Gentle Warrior

Kale, 24–26 leaves

2–4 carrots, medium

baby spinach, 1 cup arugula, 1 cup

florets and stems from 2–4 broccoli

plants 3–4 medium orange dandelion

leaves, peeled Additions that are

optional:

Replacements: Garlic and ginger, to

taste

For dandelion, use watercress.

Arugula may be substituted for romaine

lettuce. Your Mouth Is Full with

Excitement Juice 2 peeled sweet

potatoes

Carrots, 3–4

1 cayenne pepper, tiny (or cayenne

pepper powder to taste) Additions that

are optional:

Carrots, 1–2 Replacements:

Carrots for apples

The Champion's Feast 1 peeled sweet

potato a few of Roma tomatoes

medium carrots, tiny beets

florets and stems from 2–3 broccoli

plants

parsley, a handful

12 onion (white or purple) 1 tiny ginger

chunk

2 garlic cloves Additions that are

optional:

1 tiny turmeric chunk Replacements:

Broccoli with celery

To substitute an apple for a tomato,

The Enchilada in Its Entirety 3–4 kale

leaves

3–4 Romaine lettuce leaves 1 pound of

spinach

1 arugula cup

parsley, a handful

basil leaves, a handful

a sprig of dandelion 1 pineapple cup

Approximately 8–10 strawberries

1 tiny ginger chunk Additions that are

optional:

1 tiny turmeric chunk 1 pepper, jalapeo

Replacements:

Green collards may be substituted for

kale or spinach.

Rad-ish 2–3 kale leaves radish (remove

stems)

14 cucumbers (English)

4 radish bulbs, medium (with greens)

To taste, fresh ginger

14 cup of water

Peel the ginger root and squeeze out as much juice as possible, adding additional water if required.

The cucumber just slightly cools down the spiciness of the radish and ginger.

This is an excellent drink for clearing the respiratory system or for people who suffer from seasonal allergies.

When you add bee pollen to the mix, the anti-allergy benefits are double. You may also add an Asian touch by using daikon radish instead of the traditional red bulb.

Broccolean

1 tiny broccoli crown 1 parsley bunch cucumber, medium 4 carrots Juice.

Broccolean delivers your daily dosage

of veggies and helps you work your way

to a smaller shape and a healthier heart

in only one glass, making it an easier

taste for a more seasoned juice-goer.

Carrots are rich in sugar, but they also

provide your immune system a boost,

helping you fight sickness and improve

your general health. Because parsley is

high in antioxidants, it's a great all-

around beauty drink.

Blended Fruit and Vegetables

A Pineapple-Kale Blast to Remember 6–

8 big kale leaves (with stem)

12 big cucumbers (Italian)

a dozen bunches of parsley

2–212 cup peeled pineapple chunks 34–

1 cup strawberries Additions that are

optional:

Replacements: a handful of fresh mint

Any cucumber will do

Kale with Swiss chard

For the strawberries, use either a sweet

apple or pineapple, but not both The

Vitamin C Minty Rush

a third to a fourth of a cup of baby

spinach

parsley, a handful

apples, tiny and tasty

2 peeled medium oranges stems 6–8

mint leaves

a single lemon

1 tiny ginger chunk Additions that are

optional:

1–2 Persian cucumbers, tiny

Replacements:

Use all oranges or all apples in your

recipe. Dan the Dapper

4 stems Bok choy is a kind of Chinese

cabbage.

2–4 short-stemmed broccoli crowns kale

leaves, 4–6

1 cup grapes (green)

2–3 Granny Smith apples, tiny a single

lemon

Additions that are optional

1 tiny ginger chunk Alternatives:

lime in place of lemon

Kale may be substituted with spinach or

collard greens. The Emerald Deluxe

Edition

2–3 cups spinach (baby or normal)

celery stems, 3–4

3–4 tiny cucumbers from Persia 1 cup

grapes (green or red) 1 Granny Smith

apple

a tiny ginger piece Additions that are

optional:

a handful of mint or dill leaves

Replacements:

Any cucumber will do

For spinach, use collard greens or kale.

The Green Uprising

6–8 collard green leaves 1 medium cucumber from Italy

medium Granny Smith apples, a large handful of parsley 1 peeled

medium orange

tiny seedless jalapeo pepper

12 limes

Optional Additions: peeled garlic cloves

Replacements: a chunk of ginger

Any cucumber will do

For collard greens, use spinach or kale. The Elixir of Shanti Om

cilantro, a handful 2–3 celery stalks

A tiny Romaine lettuce head 4–6 Swiss chard leaves

1 red apple, tiny

1 apple, medium yellow

12 limes 1 kiwifruit

Additions that are optional:

Replacements: Garlic and ginger, to taste

Lettuce for spinach

For cilantro, use parsley.

Is there another sweet apple that might be substituted? 13 of a big

fennel, Frothy Monkey Juice

a bundle of mint leaves

Watercress, a tiny handful 4 big kale leaves

a ginger root piece 1–112 quarts pineapple Approximately 8–10 strawberries Additions that are optional:

a little amount of turmeric

1–2 garlic cloves, peeled Replacements:

Kale may be substituted with spinach or collard greens. Fennel with a pinch of dill or mint

The Goddess of the Green 37–38 kale leaves, big

12–2 cups spinach (baby or normal) a dozen strawberries

Medium–large Granny Smith apple

mint leaves, a handful

14 bulb and stem of fennel a single lime

Additions that are optional

a smattering of dill substitutes:

For lime, use lemon.

For mint, use cilantro or parsley. The Comforting Feeling

3–4 big Swiss chard leaves 3–4 broccoli stalks and florets

a few sprigs of parsley

12 big cucumbers (Italian) a single lemon

Approximately 6–8 strawberries

apples from a tiny orchard Additions that are optional:

1–2 garlic cloves, peeled 2–4 basil leaves Replacements:

Any cucumber will do

Any other apple that is delicious

For Swiss chard, use spinach or kale.

The Dragonfly of Zen

2–3 cups spinach (baby or normal) A tiny Romaine lettuce head 1 medium Granny Smith apple 1 medium pear Approximately 8–10 strawberries

Additions that are optional:

Replacements: ginger and garlic to taste

Strawberry substitute: raspberries Pears can be substituted for apples and vice versa. The Emerald Dream

1 peeled grapefruit

1 peeled orange

1 apple, Honey Crisp (or any other) 2 fennel stalks and 14 bulb

12 basil bunch

12 c. cilantro

1 large cucumber from Italy

tiny piece of raw turmeric Additions that are optional:

Replacements: ginger and garlic to taste

Any cucumber will do

All grapefruit or all orange

The Unbelievably Creamy Lush Dream 1 large sweet potato, peeled\smedium red apples 3–4 medium size carrots Additions that are optional:

jalapeño pepper, seedless Replacements:

Any other apple that is delicious Cayenne pepper for jalapeño

The Perfect Simple Essence

Roma or other type tomatoes Carrots, 3–4

1 small yellow or red sweet bell pepper, seedless 2 Persian cucumbers

1 tiny ginger chunk Additions that are optional:

1 handful of parsley 1 clove garlic, peeled Replacements:

Any cucumber will do The Sexy Sassy Surprise Carrots, 3–4

1 medium head of Romaine lettuce Approximately 8–10 strawberries

1 medium or large pear 1 handful of fresh basil

½–1 lime

Additions that are optional:

1–2 garlic cloves, peeled Replacements:

Any other lettuce except iceberg

For lime, use lemon.

Mint or fennel for basil The Yellow Sunset

2–2½ cups Baby or regular spinach

¼ fennel bulb and stalk 2 small oranges, peeled\s1–1½ cups mango,

peeled Additions that are optional:

A handful of fresh mint or basil Replacements:

Apple for mango Cool Slaw

1 crown broccoli\s½ small red cabbage 2 carrots

1 lemon (peeled)\s1 green apple

Ginger to taste

Peel ginger root and juice all. Serve over ice.

A fresh-tasting summer delight perfect for parties by the pool,

barbecues, and picnics at the park. Besides being the ideal

accompaniment to any afternoon outside, Cool Slaw brings a lot to

the picnic table.

Broccoli's cancer-fighting properties combat the carcinogens introduced to your meat from that smokey grill. Ginger works to settle stomachs and has long been a remedy for heartburn from those summer snacks. Serve with a few extra apples in your favourite punch bowl.

The Tummy Rub

This green juice is an efficient cleanser and tonic of the hardworking yet delicate digestive system. Drink it half an hour before a heavy meal, as it stimulates your gut and gets it ready for action. You can also replace a meal with it if you're feeling heavy from a previous binge.

1 cup pineapple chunks

½ fennel bulb

½ cucumber 1 cup spinach\s½ lemon

Process all the ingredients in a juicer and serve.

Fennel has an aniseed flavour and, similar to that seed, aids digestion and prevents gas. It is also known to be a diuretic, reduce inflammation, and prevent cancer. As a food, only the round bulb is usually used, but for juicing use the bulb, stalks, and leaves. Everything goes.

4 Carrot Gold

4 carrots

2 large kale leaves 1 bok choy bulb\sgolden apple

Ginger to taste

Peel ginger root and juice all. Serve over ice.

Rich, I say, rich! Rich in vitamins, colour, and in flavour, that is. Adding apple has always been a great way to balance out the grainy sweetness of carrots and still deliver the unbeatable shot of beta-carotene you get from them.

Bok choy's health-promoting compounds are better preserved when it is left uncooked, and what better way to maximise these rich health benefits. Break out the blender and have yourself a gold rush.

Red Queen\skale leaves

1 medium beet

1 gala apple\s¼ red cabbage

1 bunch red grapes Juice.

Long live the queen. Super sweet, sassy, and deep, dark red, Red Queen is one smart drink. Grape juice promotes brain health and memory function. Red cabbage is rich in iodine, which also promotes proper brain and nervous system function. One sip and you'll be singing the Red Queen's "Off with the cabbage head!" Just remember what the dormouse said, "Feed your head!"

Beetle Juice

1 yellow bell pepper 1 Fuji apple

1 small crown broccoli 1 small beet

½ sweet potato\shandful parsley\scarrots Juice.

Saying it three times in succession may not raise the dead, but it will certainly raise your spirits and your energy levels. Bell pepper is a natural immune booster and coupled with broccoli, you've got yourself one helluva free- radical fighter. Eating sweet root vegetables like beets and sweet potato helps calm sugar cravings, so put down that donut and drink your veggies.

Hot Rocket

2 Gala apples

2 handfuls of arugula 1 handful of cilantro

2 cups coconut water/milk

1 smidgen of jalapeño (to taste) (to taste)

Soy sauce to taste

Juice and mix with coconut water and soy sauce.

This one is a bit different. We've got very bold and spicy flavours here. The coconut water, jalapeño, and salty soy sauce combine to give Hot Rocket a kind of Thai flavour while the cilantro brings back the Mexican flare.

Cilantro is also great for removing heavy metals from the bloodstream and jalapeños can raise your body temperature thereby increasing your metabolic rate. The healthy fats in the coconut milk will allow increase in mineral absorption from the arugula and cilantro.

Dande-Lemon

1 bunch dandelion greens 1 bulb radicchio

Ginger to taste\s1 lemon (juiced, to taste) (juiced, to taste)

Dash cayenne\sJuice and mix in cayenne.

The ginger, lemon, and cayenne do a great job of taming the bitterness of the blood-and liver-purifying dandelion greens. This is like a suped-up lemonade. Master Cleanse aficionados will appreciate the lemon juice–cayenne pairing, which increases your body's fat-burning power and strengthens your immune system. Not much else to say except, it's really dandy.

Veggie-All\sbeet\sstalks celery

1 green bell pepper 1 large cucumber

Lemon (juiced, to taste) (juiced, to taste) 1 tsp olive oil

Juice and mix (shake) with olive oil.

Olive oil is a phytonutrient powerhouse and also helps the body absorb the many vitamins and minerals in the other vegetables.

You might want to play with the amount of green bell pepper here because sometimes the flavour can completely take over, or perhaps use a yellow or red pepper since they have a fruitier flavour.

Sometimes I even add a couple of carrots to sweeten the lot.

Green King

1 crown broccoli

1 green apple\sbunch green grapes 2 handfuls spinach\slarge leaves collard greens Juice.

Where would we be without a solid green drink? I introduce you to a king and his crown . . . of broccoli?

Absolutely. Broccoli, the miracle food, packs the most nutritional punch of any vegetable, and it meets your complete fibre need providing both soluble and insoluble fibre. Green grapes are a natural antihistamine and despite their tiny stature, they really add quite a bit of sweetness. A juice fit for a king.

Rocket Fuel

2 oz. (juiced) wheatgrass (or kale) (or kale) 2 handfuls arugula

1–2 oranges (peeled) Juice.

All the energy and alertness provided by a shot of espresso without the shakes and eventual crash—this is what you can find in wheatgrass.

Wheatgrass is a high-alkaline, nutritionally dense green with a fairly potent flavour that some people have a hard time acclimating to; that's why you'll often find it paired with fresh orange slices at your local fresh juice bar. Not to mention it infuses the already high vitamin content with a significant amount of immune-boosting Vitamin C.

Green Clean

a single lime

a single lemon

1 large cucumber

1 handful basil\shandful mint\shandfuls spinach

Ginger to taste Juice.

This one begs to be put into a giant ice-filled punch bowl and ladled into frosty glasses poolside. You'll never know your body is detoxifying as you gulp this delicious summer treat. Some folks may find it a bit too sour, so try adding an apple or two if that's the case.

Not only do we have great flavour, high amounts of vitamins, minerals, and antioxidants, Green Clean is one of the most aromatically appealing drinks in this book. Crisp, clean, refreshing.

Ginger Snap

3–4 handfuls spinach 1 small anise bulb

Ginger to taste 3–4 dates

cup frozen cherries (optional) (optional)

Juice spinach, anise, and ginger. Toss in a blender with dates and, for a Ginger Roy Rogers, add cherries. Blend. Serve over ice.

This is practically a liquid dessert. Anise is great for digestion and paired with ginger, this drink is a perfect after-meal delight. The anise has a sophisticated licorice flavour that when paired with the sweetness of the dates makes for a dreamy combination.

The ginger adds a nice bite that helps steer you away from diabetic shock. Throw in a few frozen cherries to brighten it up or dare I say, add a scoop of sugar-free coconut ice cream for a float you won't soon forget.

Blimey Mary!

medium tomatoes

2 celery stalks

1 bunch watercress

1–2 green onions (to taste) (to taste) Carrots, 1–2

1 lime (peeled) (peeled)

Tabasco and pepper to taste Juice. Add Tabasco and pepper.

A more savoury flavour profile, the Blimey has heat, spice, and a double shot of nutrients. Celery, known as the zero-calorie vegetable, yields a sweet, savoury, and slightly salty taste while the watercress and green onion spice it up a bit.

Tomatoes, the highlight of this drink, accounts for the slight sweet flavour and contains high levels of lycopene, known to fight against a list of cancers.

Add a dash of Tabasco for an extra kick and you've got a simple way to get that tomato juice taste without adding an unnecessary amount of sodium to your diet.

Cold Killah

3–4 leaves purple kale 1 lemon (peeled) (peeled)

Ginger to taste 1 clove garlic

45–50 drops echinacea

2–3 carrots\ssweet red bell pepper

Juice. Add echinacea and mix.

Packed with Vitamin C, Cold Killah is the perfect cure or preemptive strike during cold season. Not only is echinacea known to boost the immune system, but so does the high amount of beta-carotene from both the carrots and red bell pepper.

Juicing to fight colds and illness is always a healthier and tastier alternative to those powdered cure packets any day. Sensing that tickle in your throat? Juice up a batch of Cold Killah, it'll stop that cold bug in its tracks.

Gold 'n' Delicious\sGolden Delicious apples 1 kiwi (peeled) (peeled)

2 cups chopped mustard greens 2 stalks celery

1 peach (pitted) (pitted) Juice.

Another dark green with heavy cancer-fighting properties, mustard greens have a spicier flavour profile than most others in the cruciferous family. Though these greens are often cooked, when juiced, their health benefits are amplified.

Toss in some sweet apples, peach, and kiwi to cut the spice and add a dose of vitamins and antioxidants and you've got yourself one delicious drink.

Blues beetle

If you grew up in the 1980s, the hue of this juice may remind you of grape-flavored chewing gum rolls in hard plastic containers. Thankfully, the bright colour is the product of all the nutrition contained inside blueberries and beets, rather than frightening chemicals and colorings.

a single beet (with leaves, optional) 1 pound of blueberries

12 romaine lettuce romaine lettuce romaine lettuce romaine lettuce romaine lettuce 2 ribs of celery

a dozen cucumbers

12 apples

12–1 inch piece peeled ginger

In a juicer, combine all of the ingredients and serve.

When cooking with beets, don't throw away the greens. They're just as tasty as the roots and have the same earthy taste. Beets were first cultivated for their leaves, not for their roots. Beets may be yellow or white, but nothing beats the deep magenta hue that normal beets provide to any beverage.

Woman of Pink Magic

Every time you drink a glass of this juice, the colour is so beautiful and vivid that it seems like you're sipping an elixir of youth and beauty. You may add freshly squeezed orange juice, or replace the strawberries with raspberries for a more acidic flavour, in addition to adding ginger to give it a spicy and warming sensation.

1 cup strawberries (beets)

12 romaine lettuce romaine lettuce romaine lettuce romaine lettuce romaine lettuce

a dozen cucumbers

12 inch ginger root, peeled

In a juicer, puree the ingredients and serve.

Beets should be included in your diet as often as possible, particularly during the winter months when they are in season. However, due of their high sugar content, they should not be consumed in excess. The same applies for carrots and sweeter fruits: a little amount, used often, goes a long way.

Dandelion Beet-er

This brightly colourful and flavorful juice isn't for the faint of heart. Although the bitterness of dandelion may turn off sweetness lovers, I find that its excellent cleansing qualities more than compensate for it. There is no gain without suffering.

leaves of dandelion

a single beet

12 cucumbers 1 carrot

1 lemon (12–1)

12 apple Granny Smith (optional) Combine all of the ingredients in a juicer and serve.

If you want a really extreme version of this drink, leave the apple out. The sugar content of the beets and carrots is already high, and adding additional fruit would just increase it. If you truly need it, though, you may add the fruit to get the advantages.

past your taste senses with dandelion leaves

Vegetables Must Be Saved

This juice was originally made to use up some leftover tomatoes and spinach that had been sitting in the fridge for a few days. These vegetables took a 180o turn thanks to the sweetness provided by the berries and pineapple water.

1 pound of berries

a single tomato

spinach, 1–2 cups

1–2 cup pineapple juice

The first three components should be juiced.

Combine the pineapple juice with the pineapple water and serve.

Tomatoes are a member of the nightshades family of foods, which have a poor reputation due to the presence of chemicals that induce inflammation and discomfort. Nightshades, which include potatoes, peppers, and eggplants, are defended by proponents who argue that the advantages much exceed any possible harm produced by such tiny quantities of these poisons. What's our conclusion? You can get good results from almost everything as long as you don't overdo it.

Young Forever

The sweetness of the carrots and the acidity of the lemon in this delightful juice nicely complement the strong cilantro taste. As a consequence, you'll have a delicious drink that will help you get rid of a lot of pollutants. This is a dish you'll want to make again and again, not just because it's good for your liver, but also because it's good for you.

a dozen cucumbers 1 carrot, big

1 cup coriander 12 lemon juice

Cucumber, carrots, and cilantro should all be juiced. Squeeze the lemon and mix it into the juice.

When it's hot and humid outdoors, who needs a cool beer? This juice's minerals will satisfy your thirst better than any other beverage.

Lettuce Rest

Because both apples and lettuce are very soothing, this tranquil elixir is an excellent pre-sleep breakfast or snack. In one drink, the components in this juice will keep you satisfied, slim your waistline, and aid liver detoxification.

Good luck with your snoozing!

1 apple, Granny Smith

a dozen cucumbers

1 head of romaine lettuce

4 sprigs of mint

12 limes

In a juicer, combine all of the ingredients and serve.

Instead of splitting the lettuce head in half, start peeling layers from the outside in when you're not going to utilise the whole head. This will prevent it from browning where the cut is made. Refrigerate it in an airtight plastic bag.

PROBIOTIC DRINK PART IV

Recipes for Komucha

Kombucha is a fermented tea.

Kombucha is a probiotic beverage that is inherently bubbling (or "effervescent"). It began in Northeast China and eventually made its way to Russia. After then, Kombucha was introduced to Germany, followed by the rest of Europe and the rest of the globe. Kombucha is produced from a SCOBY (Symbiotic Culture of Bacteria and Yeast), which is a live creature. A SCOBY is also known as "the mother" or "mushroom." It multiplies, ferments, and feeds on tea and sugar as it grows and multiplies. The bacteria and yeast consume the sugar, causing the beverage to ferment and produce an acidic, probiotic-rich, and slightly alcoholic beverage. When fermenting live organisms, like with all of the recipes in this book, care is advised.

Acetic acid, found in kombucha, is a moderate natural antibacterial. Bad bacteria strains cannot develop in kombucha cultures due to the acidity, since the environment is not conducive to survival or reproduction. The beneficial bacteria flourish in this environment, whereas the harmful bacteria have little chance of surviving. Kombucha is also high in B vitamins, folate, and antioxidants, as well as lactic acid.

Kombucha is said to help with digestion, energy, appetite

management, and restoring pH balance in the digestive system. There is still a lot of dispute about whether these health claims are backed up by scientific evidence. It's essential to remember that this book doesn't promise drinking kombucha will enhance your health, and that the claimed advantages won't apply to everyone. Regardless, kombucha tastes wonderful, and most people say it helps them feel better by regulating their digestive tract.

If you've ever bought kombucha or any other probiotic beverage from the supermarket, you've probably noticed how pricey it is. I started making kombucha because I was always drinking store-bought kombucha and the price was getting out of hand for my budget. I started brewing kombucha with a few modest start-up expenses, and it's been an investment that's paid for itself hundreds of times over.

At first, brewing kombucha may seem overwhelming and frightening, but don't be fooled by the lengthy list of instructions. Making homemade kombucha is really very simple, but I want to stress the necessity of brewing properly by giving comprehensive instructions.

How to Begin

You'll need various kitchen equipment, as well as a kombucha SCOBY in starting liquid, to make kombucha. Homebrewed kombucha is used as the starter liquid. A SCOBY may be purchased from a variety of internet sites. Because the quality of certain SCOBY vendors is more trustworthy than others, I advise you to study reviews and speak with people who have bought from the particular suppliers you are considering. If you buy your SCOBY online, make sure you start brewing as soon as possible since the SCOBY will be in a state of shock from the journey, and it's critical to keep it nourished and in a healthy environment as soon as possible.

Maintaining the Health of Your SCOBY and Kombucha

What does it take to keep a SCOBY alive and well? I'll mention it a few times throughout the list of instructions, but it basically means: 1. Feeding the SCOBY a tea and sugar combination; the ideal tea for making kombucha is 100 percent black tea, but you may also use 100 percent green tea. Fancy teas often include peels and other components that are incompatible with kombucha fermentation. It's best to use plain black tea.

Keeping it dark and out of the sun: a closet shelf is a great location to keep kombucha or jun fermenting.

A kitchen towel or cheesecloth fastened by a flexible rubber band works wonderfully to keep the pests out while yet allowing it to breathe.

Keeping it at a comfortable temperature (between 75 and 85 degrees Fahrenheit).

Using starting liquid to keep the SCOBY wet. For every inch of SCOBY, I suggest keeping at least two inches of starting liquid.

If you get your SCOBY online, make sure you start brewing a batch as soon as possible since the SCOBY will be shocked.

Giving Away One of Your SCOBYs

A fresh SCOBY will develop with each each batch of kombucha you make. While it's OK to let the SCOBY develop, I feel that my SCOBY looks the healthiest when it's three inches thick or less. Layers of your kombucha SCOBY may be peeled off and given to friends or family.

To do so, fill a plastic bag halfway with starting liquid (kombucha) and a SCOBY. When transporting the SCOBY, ensure sure it is properly sealed and that it is kept level and out of direct sunlight.

Because the SCOBY will be in shock from the trip, it is critical that it be taken out of the bag as soon as possible so it can breathe. Tell the person you're giving the SCOBY to make a batch of kombucha as soon as possible.

They bring the SCOBY back to their house.

Kombucha fermentation

There must be food for the active probiotics and yeasts to feed on, just as in any other fermentation process. Food for kombucha is tea and sugar. A new SCOBY will develop with each batch of kombucha you make, and the SCOBY will expand to the breadth of the container it is in. When you make your fifth batch of kombucha, for example, you'll have five layers of SCOBY. You may let your SCOBY develop while you brew, and you don't have to discard it until it's more than three inches thick.

Kombucha, in addition to tea and sugar, needs a certain temperature range to thrive. The ideal temperature range for brewing kombucha is between 75° and 85° Fahrenheit. While temperatures outside of that range are usually OK for kombucha, you will notice a difference in the intensity of the kombucha if it is brewed below 70° or over 80°. A lower temperature may need more brewing time, while a higher temperature may accelerate the fermentation process. The probiotics may be killed if the temperature is too high.

Flavoring kombucha is one of the most enjoyable aspects of the process. It's absolutely acceptable to consume your kombucha straight from the bottle without putting it through a secondary fermentation; but, for the sake of your kombucha pleasure, I've included many recipes for making bubbly, sweet kombucha that may be enjoyed all year. It's important to note that flavoured kombucha should be added after the initial fermentation, since anything other than sweetened tea in a SCOBY's environment may alter the structure and health of the bacteria.

Secondary Fermentation: What Is It and How Does It Work?

Secondary fermentation refers to the process of fermenting a beverage that has already been fermented once. The bacteria and yeast in kombucha feed on the sugar and tea you give them during the initial fermentation. The probiotics are ready for more after they have eaten all of the "meal." Secondary fermentation is used in this case.

You may start a secondary fermentation right after the initial fermentation (but before you refrigerate the kombucha) by adding more tea and water. You may also flavour your kombucha with a variety of fruits, herbs, and non-toxic flowers. After you've added the extra ingredients, bottle the kombucha and store it in a dark, room-temperature location for two to three days to continue fermenting.

Because the bottles are sealed, some pressure will build up, causing the liquid to fizz (or naturally carbonated). The more sugar you add, the longer it will take the probiotics to ferment, much like the initial fermentation.

it's being processed If you want your kombucha to be sweeter, either add more sugar (cane sugar or fruit) than is required, or limit the second fermentation to one or two days rather than two to three. When you refrigerate kombucha, fermentation slows but does not cease entirely.

Now here comes the really cool part! Depending on what you use for the secondary fermentation, you will end up with varying levels of effervescence. I found that more acidic fruit yields a more effervescent kombucha. I have also found that leaving fruit pulp inside the bottles during the secondary fermentation results in more effervescence. Additionally, allowing the sealed bottles to refrigerate for at least twenty-four hours before popping the bottle open will yield a more effervescent kombucha.

To summarise: to get the most effervescent kombucha (if that is what you're going for), use an acidic fruit for the secondary fermentation process, leaving the pulp inside the bottles and allowing the bottles to sit for two to three days at room temperature. Then refrigerate the bottles for one to two days before drinking. Berries, apricots, and pineapple have resulted in the spunkiest kombucha in my experience. Remember to shorten the length of the secondary fermentation if you desire a sweeter (less dry) kombucha.

Because pressure and effervescence builds during the secondary fermentation, it is very important that you point the bottles away from your face when you open them. If you are using good quality flip-cap bottles, it is likely that you will have a batch or two of kombucha that will fizz out of the bottle when opened, similar to opening a can of soda after it's been rolling around in the back of your car). Just be sure to open the bottles over the sink and never point them at your face or anything breakable. Do not ever give a small child a bottle of kombucha to open.

Kombucha and Allergies and/or Detox

A very small portion of the population is allergic to kombucha. The exact science behind the allergy is unknown. Similar to doing a juice cleanse, some people go through a detoxification after drinking kombucha. This may be perceived as an allergic reaction but it could be the body ridding itself of toxins. Symptoms of detox include headache, more frequent than usual bowel movements, runny nose, or even vomiting. Should you experience any of these symptoms, it is best to consult a doctor before attempting to consume any more kombucha.

It is not recommended to drink homemade kombucha on an empty stomach. If your stomach ever hurts after drinking kombucha, it could mean one of three things—your batch is bad (unlikely, unless you notice mould and/or the batch tastes abnormal), you drank too much, or your kombucha is too strong.

Depending on the ingredients added for secondary fermentation, it is possible for people to have a negative reaction to one flavour and have no problem with other flavours.

Taking a Break Between Batches of Kombucha

By no means do you have to continue brewing kombucha forever and ever with no break between batches. Once your SCOBY is growing, you may consider peeling off one of the SCOBYs and using it in an additional jug to brew a higher volume of kombucha at one time. With that said, you may end up with more kombucha than you feel you need or you may simply get sick of brewing. Never fear, you don't have to throw your kombucha SCOBY out! You can store your kombucha

SCOBY in the same way you would store kombucha that is brewing: in a jar covered with cheesecloth bound with a rubber band.

Be sure there is plenty of starter fluid to keep the SCOBY moist. One inch of starter fluid for every one inch of SCOBY works well. You will need this starter fluid to keep your SCOBY alive and also to start your next batch when you are ready to brew again. If you go several weeks between batches, check on the SCOBY every once in a while to be sure it still has ample starter fluid.

Cleaning Your Tools

It is very important that everything you use that touches the SCOBY and/or kombucha be properly sanitised. You can sanitise your tools in the dishwasher, or with hot, soapy water, or by soaking them in distilled white vinegar for a couple minutes. If there is harmful bacteria on any of the tools you use, it can potentially contaminate your kombucha.

You do not need to clean the jug that you use to brew kombucha between batches. I do, however, recommend that you clean it periodically (I clean mine every three to five batches) (I clean mine every three to five batches). To clean the jug, pour all of the kombucha liquid into bottles (if you haven't already) except for a small amount of fluid to act as starter for your next batch. Place the SCOBY and starter fluid into a glass or stainless steel bowl and cover with a kitchen towel. Fill the jug with very hot, soapy water and use a sponge to get every last bit of kombucha culture out. I repeat this process multiple times to ensure my jug is sanitary.

Distilled white vinegar acts as a sanitising agent, so you can use vinegar to clean the jug, as well. Pour about ½ cup of distilled white vinegar in the jug and slosh it around for a minute or two. Pour the vinegar out. You can either rinse the jug with clean spring/well water or simply leave it as is. A little bit of residual vinegar will not harm your SCOBY.

Now you can start another batch of kombucha by first adding your tea/sugar mixture to the jug and then carefully (and with clean hands) pouring the starter liquid and SCOBY back in the jug. Secure the opening with cheesecloth bound by a rubber band.

Flavoring Your Kombucha

While it is not necessary to add flavours to kombucha once it has finished its primary fermentation, experimenting with flavours is by far the most fun part of brewing kombucha! There are a myriad of options for giving your kombucha flavour, spunk, and fizz. Fresh fruit and herbs are my favourite ingredients to add before secondary fermentation to ensure the beverage will be bubbly, just the right amount of sweetness, and full of added health benefits.

One-hundred percent fruit juices are also effective for secondary fermentation, although not to the same extent as fresh fruit. Kombucha likes fruit pulp and tends to be much fizzier when fruit pulp is added for secondary fermentation. For every one gallon of kombucha, 1 cup of fruit juice can be added for secondary fermentation.

It is important to be mindful of the strength of your kombucha. If your kombucha is strong (meaning its pH is lower than 2.5), dilute it with additional sweetened tea along with fruit or other ingredients prior to the secondary fermentation. This ensures there will be enough sugar and tea for the probiotics to feed on for an effective secondary fermentation and will also ensure the kombucha is safe for consumption.

Typically for a gallon of strong kombucha, steeping 4

teabags in 4 cups of water and adding some sugar (¼ to ½ cup) is sufficient to dilute it, but depending on the strength, a higher amount of freshly brewed tea may be used. Always cool the tea (and any other hot ingredients) to room temperature before mixing it with kombucha because excessive heat will kill the probiotics.

Because you will need to save starter liquid (for every one inch of SCOBY, I typically save one to two inches of starter liquid) and also to leave some room at the top of the jar so that the liquid doesn't spill over when the jar is moved, you will not get a true gallon when brewing 1 gallon of kombucha. The liquid yield is closer to ¾ gallon or less depending on how thick your SCOBY is. Similarly, when brewing kombucha in a 2-gallon jug, you will not get a full 2 gallons of kombucha. Most individuals brew either 1 gallon or 2 gallons of kombucha at a time, so I chose to focus my kombucha recipes on the 1-gallon batches. This means each recipe in this section calls for ¾ gallon of kombucha, but you can easily double the recipes if desired.

Don't Be Surprised If . . .

Don't be surprised when small SCOBYs form in the bottles during secondary fermentation. Because the probiotics and yeast continue to ferment, they form a colony during secondary fermentation, which is clear, gooey, and typically the size of a quarter. If you drink one by accident, nothing bad will happen, although the slimy texture going down your throat is not desirable for most people. Prior to drinking kombucha, use a fine strainer to catch whatever bacteria and yeast colonies (and/or fruit pulp that was added for flavor) have formed so that you can enjoy a SCOBY-free beverage.

- If your SCOBY develops lengthy brown threads beneath it, don't be shocked. These are yeast colonies that resemble kelp in appearance. They are quite normal and do not need cleaning or removal. Some people erroneously believe that these furry-looking threads indicate that the SCOBY has gone bad when, in fact, they indicate that the SCOBY is healthy.

- A Safety Reminder

- If you're not cautious, making homemade kombucha may be dangerous. If you're new to brewing kombucha, it's a good idea to learn as much as you can about the procedure. It's critical to maintain all of the equipment used in the kombucha-making process clean, as well as the SCOBY alive and well. It's also essential to avoid keeping kombucha in ceramic or plastic containers.

- Use common judgement and be aware that fermentation has a risk. Throw away the whole SCOBY, dump all kombucha juice, and thoroughly sterilise the jar or jug you used to brew if you detect a single trace of mould. Kombucha mould resembles bread mould in appearance: it's typically round, white or green, and fuzzy. I've brewed dozens of batches of kombucha and left my SCOBYs in their starting liquid for months at a time without ever seeing mould. Have confidence that your SCOBY will be safe as long as you follow the directions and maintain it in a healthy atmosphere.

- Before consuming kombucha, women who are breastfeeding or pregnant should contact their physicians.

Children under the age of six should not consume kombucha due to its acidic and somewhat alcoholic character. Children above the age of six may consume modest amounts of kombucha.

- Before beginning a batch of kombucha, please read the instructions thoroughly. If you bought your SCOBY online, there was probably a set of instructions included in the box. You may probably trust their directions, but just in case, read my instructions as well.

- Kombucha should never have a bad odour or flavour. It should have a somewhat sweet but vinegary flavour, as well as a similar aroma. Because homebrewed kombucha is considerably stronger than store-bought kombucha, the aroma and flavour will be much stronger. This is very normal. If a rotten odour develops or the taste does not set well in your tongue, discard the whole batch and start again with a new SCOBY.

- Drinking homemade kombucha may get so powerful that it tastes like vinegar. Kombucha's ideal pH is between 2.5 to 4.5, which is on the acidic side. Kombucha's acidic pH prevents it from fermenting.

-

- strewn with pathogenic bacteria A pH of less than 2.5 is considered too acidic for human consumption and must be diluted before ingestion. If your kombucha's pH falls below 2.5, add additional tea and sugar and test it again before bottling. A pH greater than 4.5 creates an ideal environment for harmful bacteria to thrive.

- While it is completely safe to consume kombucha on a daily basis, most experts advise not exceeding 6 to 8 ounces of homebrewed kombucha each day. Commercially produced kombucha is subjected to many controls and testing, making it safe to consume in greater quantities. Because most individuals who make kombucha (including me) don't have sophisticated pH- and bacteria-testing equipment, it's best to drink less to avoid disturbing your digestive system's equilibrium.

- You may purchase pH test strips to obtain a rough sense of how strong your kombucha is if you're worried about maintaining a certain pH level in your kombucha. Because pH test strips may provide confusing results, you'll need to purchase a pH tester to get a more precise measurement. Although it is not essential to test the pH of every batch of kombucha, I do suggest doing so on a regular basis, particularly if you suspect your kombucha is getting too strong.

- If you've made a batch of faulty kombucha and are experiencing unpleasant side effects, see a doctor right once. Always, ALWAYS toss everything away and start again when in doubt. It's unlikely that a poor batch will occur if the SCOBY you use to start your first batch of kombucha is healthy and you follow the guidelines. However, poor kombucha may have severe side effects, so be cautious.

- Have fun with your kombucha that you made yourself!

-

- Kombucha's active probiotics and yeasts get their energy from tea and sugar.

- Kombucha Basics:

- Ingredients (about 1 gallon of kombucha):

- 1 cup of kombucha 1 (scant) gallon spring or well water SCOBY Use bottled water instead of tap water since it is likely to include chlorine and/or fluoride.

- 10 tea bags (no frills) black or green tea

- * 1 cup cane sugar *Make sure you use 100 percent black or 100 percent green tea. Many businesses use orange peel in black tea because it contains essential oils that are bad for brewing. For the greatest effects, stick to 100 percent pure teas.

-

- You'll also require:

- Large water-boiling pot

- Large glass jug/container (1 gallon or more) for fermenting the kombucha

- Stirring spoon with a long handle

- Floating or stick-on thermometer

- breathable dish towel or cheesecloth

- Rubber band that stretches

- • Small fine filter • Glass pitcher or other effective means of transporting kombucha from the jug to bottles or the dispenser you'll be drinking it from (we use a metal coffee strainer)

- Bottles made of glass with resealable closures. Screw-top and flip-cap bottles also work, although dark glass is preferred since kombucha does not like sunshine.

-

- Before boiling, add water to a sanitised pot.

- While brewing, cover your jug with cheesecloth to enable the kombucha to breathe.

- Optional Resources:

- Cleaning your kombucha container with distilled white vinegar

- An electric heating pad is an example of a heating gadget. If your home is chilly throughout the winter, they are excellent for keeping the temperature of your kombucha stable.

- Blanket for outer space. It's possible to utilise it to keep heat in. Wrapping the kombucha jug in a heating pad and securing it with a space blanket works wonderfully during chilly periods.

- How to brew kombucha at home:

- Sanitize all of the equipment you'll be using to brew kombucha. You may accomplish this by putting it in the dishwasher, hand-washing it with detergent in extremely hot water, or covering it with distilled white vinegar.

- Bring water to a boil. You don't need to boil the whole gallon of kombucha to brew the tea—just enough (12 gallon or so) to make the tea. This manner, after the tea is made, you may add the leftover water to chill it down.

- Remove the water from the heat after it has reached a boil and add the tea bags. Remove the tea bags after 8 to 10 minutes of steeping.

- Stir in the cane sugar until it dissolves completely.

- Allow the tea to cool to a temperature of 75 to 85 degrees Fahrenheit (or if you only boiled half a gallon of water, add the remaining half gallon of cool water so that the hot water cools faster).

-

- When the tea has reached the ideal temperature, add the SCOBY (if this is your first time making kombucha and you bought your SCOBY online, simply remove it from its package and slip it in).

- Stick a sticky thermometer to the exterior of the container if you have one that can be attached to a surface (optional).

- Cheesecloth should be used to cover the jug so that the kombucha may breathe.

- Using a flexible rubber band, secure the cheesecloth.

- Place the jug in a dark, warm location (closet) where it will not be disturbed by humans or light.

- Allow five to seven days for kombucha to brew (the longer it brews, the more sugar it eats and the stronger it is).

- Check the temperature of the kombucha on a regular basis. It should be kept between 70 and 85 degrees Fahrenheit for optimum effects. It's not a big issue if the temperature drops below 70°; the kombucha will simply take longer to brew. The probiotics may perish if the kombucha temperature rises beyond 85°F. If mould appears (it will resemble bread mould, with green/white fuzzy rings), remove the SCOBY and the whole batch of kombucha.

- Remove the cheesecloth once your kombucha is ready. NOTE: Your SCOBY will expand to the breadth of the container it's in, and a second SCOBY will develop as a result. SCOBYs will continue to grow indefinitely. When a SCOBY reaches a thickness of a couple of inches, I suggest peeling off a layer or two and discarding it or giving it to a friend along with some starting liquid so they may brew their own kombucha.

- After the initial fermentation is complete, you may either bottle your kombucha and call it a day or add items to it using the methods in this book. I find that pouring the kombucha drink from the jug into a smaller pitcher is the most convenient method. It's simple to pour the kombucha into bottles using the pitcher.

- You may either take a break and keep your SCOBY and starting liquid in the jug wrapped with cheesecloth tied with a rubber band, or you can brew a fresh batch once you've bottled the kombucha. SCOBYs may sit for months between batches as long as they are kept in a healthy environment. When taking a break, just store the jug in a warm, dark location that isn't often disturbed (just as you would if you were brewing a batch), and check the SCOBY before brewing a fresh batch, particularly if it has been resting for more than a few weeks. I usually reserve approximately two inches of starting liquid for every inch of SCOBY.

- Follow the preparation directions and keep the bottles of flavoured komucha at room temperature if you want to add items for a secondary fermentation.

-

- temperature for two to three days in a dark location The bacteria and yeast cultures consume the sugar you supplied (fructose from the juice or cane sugar) and continue to ferment throughout this process. This makes the kombucha a bit stronger and bubbly (the industry calls it "effervescent"). It's worth noting that during the secondary fermentation, a tiny SCOBY will develop in each bottle, which may be filtered out before consuming.

- Refrigerate kombucha for at least twenty-four hours before drinking for optimum effects. The lower temperature will reduce the fermentation (but the kombucha will continue to ferment), and refrigerating the kombucha will help it last longer.

Instructions

Combine the juice and kombucha in a large pitcher or container and mix thoroughly.

Fill sealable bottles halfway with pomegranate kombucha and store in a warm, dark location for two to three days for secondary fermentation.

To prevent secondary fermentation, chill the kombucha. Note that if you add juice to kombucha for a secondary fermentation, the outcome will not be as fizzy as if you used fresh fruit with the pulp. When texture is added to kombucha, it responds more strongly during secondary fermentation, producing in a more fizzier beverage. Adding juice is, nevertheless, delicious, healthy, and simple!

Kombucha with lemon and ginger

Having a bottle of lemon ginger kombucha on hand during cold and flu season is a great idea! Not only can kombucha help strengthen the immune system, but lemon and ginger are also effective cold remedies. Plus, the drink is delicious! When lemon and ginger are combined, they provide an almost creamy taste that soothes the bite you'd anticipate from the ingredients on their own, leaving your palette satisfied!

Ingredients:

four cups of water

3 tablespoons grated fresh ginger

3 tbsp freshly squeezed lemon juice

12 cup sugar cane

kombucha in a 34 gallon container (page 251) Instructions:

Bring the water and grated ginger to a full boil in a saucepan. Reduce the heat to medium and allow the water to bubble for approximately 5 minutes to infuse it with ginger flavour.

Remove the saucepan from the heat and whisk in the lemon juice and sugar until the sugar has dissolved.

Allow the pot to cool to room temperature before using. This will enable the taste of the ginger to pervade the tea.

Once the ginger tea has cooled, mix it with the kombucha in a pitcher or container (depending on the size of your pitcher, you may need to do this in halves).

Combine the kombucha and ginger tea and pour into glass bottles. Try to get as much ginger as possible into the bottles with the kombucha. Using a tight cap, secure the container.

Allow for secondary fermentation by keeping bottles in a warm, dark location for two to four days. Once the second ferment is finished, refrigerate the kombucha to delay the fermentation.

When ready to drink, strain the kombucha into a glass via a fine strainer to remove the ginger pulp and freshly formed SCOBY. Remove the pulp and enjoy your nutritious beverage!

Kombucha with Apples and Cinnamon

During the autumn and winter months, my favourite kombucha flavour is apple cinnamon. Warm spices and a sweet, tangy apple combine to create a comforting drink. This is a wonderful recipe to prepare in a big quantity and keep in bottles to enjoy for weeks since the ingredients are simple and easy to obtain at any grocery shop at any time of year.

Ingredients:

4 tea bags with apple taste

four cups of water

1 tsp cinnamon powder

18 tsp nutmeg powder

12 cup of sugar

dried apple rings, 3 oz (no preservatives)

(page 251) * 34 gallon kombucha

If you want to avoid preservatives, buy your dried apples from a natural food shop. Any dried fruit you add to kombucha should have a basic ingredients list, and it's worth spending a bit more to ensure the kombucha remains healthy and doesn't react negatively to extraneous chemicals or additives.

Instructions:

4 cups water, 4 cups water, 4 cups water, 4 cups water, 4 cups water, 4 cups water, 4 cups water, 4 cups water, 4 cups water, 4 cups water, 4 cups water

Remove the water from the boil and steep the apple-flavored tea bags for 5 to 8 minutes.

Stir in the sugar until it is completely dissolved.

Allow the sweetened apple tea to cool to room temperature before serving. Put it in the refrigerator or an ice bath until it reaches a lukewarm temperature to speed up the process.

Before filling each bottle with kombucha, cut apple rings in half and place two slices (one ring) in each container. The bottles must be sealed.

To enable kombucha to go through secondary fermentation, keep bottles in a warm, dark location for two to four days.

The kombucha should be kept refrigerated. When you're ready to drink, pour the liquid through a strainer.

during secondary fermentation, a tiny SCOBY developed in the bottle.

Blackberry Sage Kombucha

1.   The acidic and sweet blackberries give the kombucha a lot of life, since berries tend to make the beverage bubblier and inject a lot of flavour. The sage lends a subtle earthiness to the drink. Antioxidants and fibre abound in blackberries. They help with digestion, cardiovascular health, cancer cell protection, and neurological illness prevention, among other things. Sage is a mint-related plant with many health and medical advantages. It has anti-inflammatory properties, enhances memory, may be used as an antiseptic, aids allergic responses and insect bites, and is high in antioxidants!

2.   Ingredients:

3.   2 cups blackberries, ripe

4.   65 ounces sliced sage leaves (about 15 to 20 large sage leaves)

5.   13 cup sugar cane

6. kombucha in a 34 gallon container (page 251)

Instructions:

7. In a covered pot, cook blackberries over medium heat. Mash the blackberries with a fork as they heat up and begin to boil and soften.

8. Bring the sugar and sage to a moderate boil after the pulpy liquid has formed.

9. Reduce the heat to medium-low, cover the pot, and simmer for 15 to 20 minutes, or until the flavours have melded. Allowing the mixture to boil or simmer for too long will cause it to thicken.

10. To enable kombucha to go through secondary fermentation, keep bottles in a warm, dark location for two to four days.

11. Combine the kombucha and blackberry sage combination in a big saucepan or pitcher. Mix thoroughly, then

pour the blackberry sage kombucha, including the sage leaves and blackberry pulp, into sealable bottles. The bottles must be sealed.

12. Allow two to three days for the kombucha to go through secondary fermentation by storing it in a warm, dark location. It's worth noting that the longer the kombucha rests, the more sugar the bacteria consume, resulting in a less sweet and fizzy beverage.

13. After the secondary fermentation is finished, chill for at least 24 hours. The secondary fermentation will be slowed as a result, but the kombucha will continue to ferment and get fizzier while it stays in the refrigerator.

14. Use a tiny fine strainer to filter the kombucha when you're ready to consume it.

15.

16. During the secondary fermentation, filter away the sage

leaves, blackberry pulp, and any tiny SCOBY that has developed. Remove all of the pulp and enjoy the drink!

17. Kombucha with Jasmine

18. Although kombucha is best made with 100 percent black tea, you may use other flavoured teas for secondary fermentation. Use your favourite tea flavours and even loose tea if you want to go all out.

19. This soothing beverage has a great aroma and flavour. Jasmine tea is a naturally relaxing beverage that is renowned for reducing heart rate and calming the mood. Jasmine has been shown in studies to help reduce stroke and esophageal cancer. Jasmine tea gives kombucha a delicate, flowery taste and is a simple method to flavour it for secondary fermentation.

20. Ingredients:

21. 3 quarts liquid

22. 3 sachets of jasmine tea

23. 34 gallon kombucha 12 cup sugar (page 251)

Instructions:

24. Bring the water to a boil in a saucepan.

25. Steep for 5 to 8 minutes after adding the tea bags.

26. Stir in the sugar until it is completely dissolved.

27. Allow the jasmine tea to cool to room temperature before drinking. To expedite the procedure, place the pot of tea in an ice bath or pour the tea into a jug and chill it until it reaches a lukewarm temperature.

28. Combine the jasmine tea, kombucha, and sugar in a big pitcher or container.

29.

30. stir.

31. Fill sealable bottles halfway with jasmine kombucha and close tightly.

32. Allow two to four days in a warm, dark area to allow for

fermentation.

33.

34. fermentation in the second stage

35. After secondary fermentation, store the bottles in the refrigerator. When you're ready to drink, gently open bottles to avoid pressure buildup during secondary fermentation.

36.

37. Pineapple Kombucha is a fermented tea made from pineapples.

38. Are you searching for a sweet and bubbly kombucha? It's finally here! The addition of pineapple pieces to kombucha for secondary fermentation produces a highly effervescent beverage. The more acidic the fruits, I've discovered, the more effervescent the probiotic drinks. As a result, acidic fruits are excellent for flavouring these drinks; nevertheless, it is essential to use non-breakable bottles and to follow the manufacturer's

instructions.

39.

40. When opening the bottles after secondary fermentation, use extreme caution.

41. The pressure that develops during secondary fermentation from the pineapple is so high that the beverage overflows when opened from a flip-cap bottle, therefore screw-top bottles are suggested for bottling this recipe. With screw caps, a little amount of air is always allowed to escape, and you may release pressure by gently twisting the cap before opening. Do not give pineapple kombucha bottles to youngsters for safety reasons; they may burst all over the place and be dangerous for them to open. When carefully opening a bottle, it is advisable to keep your gaze away from it and never aim it at anybody. Any effervescent probiotic beverage in this book is the same way.

42. While pineapple kombucha necessitates a little more planning and care, it has a fantastic tropical taste and is especially pleasant in the spring and early summer when pineapples are in season!

43. 2 cups fresh pineapple, cut into 14 to 12 inch chunks

44. 34 gallon of kombucha brewed from scratch (page 251)

Instructions:

45. Distribute the diced pineapple evenly among the bottles you'll be bottling.

46. Fill the bottles with the kombucha and pineapple.

47. Place the bottles in a dark, warm location, such as a cupboard or closet.

48. Allow bottles to rest in a warm, dark area for two to three days to allow the kombucha to go through a secondary fermentation.

49. Before drinking the kombucha, keep it refrigerated for at

least 24 hours. If you leave the kombucha in the fridge for more than a day, it will get more effervescent.

50.

51.   Raspberry Mint Kombucha is a kombucha made with raspberries and mint

52.   The flavours of raspberries and mint combine to create a sweet, somewhat tangy, and refreshing beverage with a lot of flavour. To enable all of the flavours to open up and permeate, fresh raspberries are cooked with mint leaves. Raspberry mint kombucha is a refreshing drink any time of year, but especially during the summer when raspberries are plentiful.

53.   6 oz. raspberries, peeled and halved

54.   12 cup sugar 75 ounces fresh mint leaves, coarsely chopped

55.   14 cup of water

56.

57. kombucha in a 34 gallon container (page 251)

Instructions:

58. Remove the mint leaves from the stems and tear them into tiny pieces with your fingers (in half or thirds is fine).

59. In a small saucepan, cook the raspberries, mint leaves, sugar, and water over medium heat. Bring the mixture to a boil.

60. Smash the raspberries with a fork until they lose their shape.

61. Reduce the heat to medium-low and continue to gently boil for another 5 minutes to enable the mint to infuse.

62. Remove the pan from the heat and set aside to cool to room temperature. Pour it into a bowl or glass and put it in the refrigerator to speed up the process.

63. Combine the kombucha and raspberry-mint combination in a big pitcher or jug.

64. After mixing everything together, pour the kombucha

into bottles.

65. When you've reached the bottom, spoon the raspberry and mint pulp into the bottles, making sure the pulp is distributed equally.

66. To enable the kombucha to go through secondary fermentation, keep the bottles in a dark, warm location for two to four days.

67. Refrigerate for at least 24 hours before serving. The longer you wait to consume the kombucha, the fizzier it will get.

68. When you're ready to consume the kombucha, filter out the freshly created SCOBY as well as the raspberry and mint pulp using a fine sieve. Enjoy!

69.

70. Kombucha with figs

71. Adding figs to kombucha, smoothies, or even baked

products is a delicious way to get a naturally sweet treat. Because figs are rich in fructose and have a mild taste, they're a great way to add sweetness without becoming overwhelming. This kombucha is bubbly and sweet, with just "original" taste. You may expand this recipe to whatever quantity you want by using 1 fig per 16-ounce bottle. If you utilise the whole 34 gallon, you'll get 6 bottles.

72. Ingredients (about 1 gallon of kombucha):

73. 34 gallon kombucha 6 ripe figs, cut into tiny pieces (page 251) Fill each 16-ounce bottle halfway with coarsely chopped figs.

74. For secondary fermentation, seal bottles and put them in a warm, dark location for two days.

75. Refrigerate fig kombucha for at least 24 hours for the best results.

76.

77. before you eat it

78. When ready to eat, strain the fig pulp (along with the freshly created SCOBY) through a fine sieve.

Other Probiotic Drinks

More information about how to make kombucha and water kefir (Tibicos)

Tibicos (water kefir grains) are kefir grains that have been adapted to cultivate non-dairy drinks. Tibicos are transparent rather than white or creamy in appearance. You may use them to make water kefir, coconut kefir, or cider from sugar water, coconut water, or fruit juice. They have the same history and characteristics as the kefir grains discussed before. Because they may be used in the same manner as kombucha, I've included them here. Tibicos, on the other hand, may grow a drink in as little as 1–2 days, while kombucha takes 7–14 days to culture.

Kombucha is said to have originated in Northeast Asia, particularly in China's Manchurian area, although it may also have originated in Japan. Kombucha was first mentioned in Manchuria about 330 BC, according to one account, while it was first made in Japan around 415 AD, according to another. No one is certain that this refers to the fermented tea drink since a seaweed tea in the area had a similar name. Hundreds of years later, kombucha was discovered in a historical document in Russia, which may have been its birthplace.

The culture of the kombucha mother is one of a kind. It is, first and foremost, the most apparent of all SCOBYs, resembling a piece of rubber or silicon. Furthermore, while kefir and ginger beer cultures sink to the bottom of any liquid (at least until it becomes carbonated), the much larger kombucha SCOBY floats on top. It may develop to an inch or more in thickness and cover the whole surface area of the container. Bacillus coagulans is the bacterium responsible for the physical appearance of the kombucha mother (also known as Lactobacillus sporogenes). It produces a porous, rubbery mat that offers an ideal dwelling habitat for up to a dozen more yeasts and bacteria.

You may get a kombucha SCOBY from a friend who has extra culture to give, buy one online, or cultivate one from a bottle of kombucha. It's not difficult to grow your own. Begin by putting a store-bought bottle of kombucha, along with some tea and sugar, into a bigger jar or plastic container. After a few days, a white film may appear at the surface of the liquid, which you may mistake for mould at first. Each time you check it, you'll see that the film has thickened, ultimately turning into a thick mat that covers the surface of your fermenting beverage.

This flat blob is your very own kombucha mushroom, which you can use to make probiotic beverages and dishes at home. You may gently transfer the mushroom to a new container whenever you want to cultivate something new. If it becomes too large, break it up and split the pieces. You may compost it, share it with a friend, or utilise the leftover culture to brew another drink. SCOBYs that have been used include

Beneficial microbes contribute to good soil, which helps plants develop and remain healthy, therefore they're also excellent for your garden.

How to Make Kefir from Water (Using Tibicos)

Water kefir is produced by fermenting sugar water with tibicos (water kefir grains). The majority of individuals choose brown sugar, cane sugar, maple syrup, or another healthy sweetener that has more minerals than store-bought white sugar. If the cultures don't have adequate minerals, they won't be able to ferment properly. Water kefir is often made using water kefir grains (tibicos), although milk kefir grains may also be utilised.

Adding a pinch to a teaspoon of sea salt (depending on your taste) may also assist to guarantee that minerals are present. Add some chopped fruit or ginger to the ferment as another option. This will add some taste as well as a few extra minerals. But keep in mind that you'll have to separate the kefir grains from the fruit or ginger afterwards. And, after these grains have been removed, it is always feasible to add taste after the fermentation.

You may use coconut water from a young coconut instead of sugar water since it already has enough sugar and minerals and doesn't need any additional sweeteners or minerals. Coconut water and young coconuts are becoming more popular. Both may be found in a variety of health food shops as well as Latin American and Asian markets.

1 quart water kefir (or coconut water kefir)

Materials required:

1 mixing bowl, big (glass, plastic, or wood, but not metal)

2 jars of glass (quart-sized mason jars are good)

1 wooden spoon or silicon spatula

1 strainer made of plastic

For the jar, use cheesecloth, a towel, or a sprouting lid. 1 quart of filtered (nonchlorinated) water or coconut water (young)

14 cup water kefir grains (4 tbsp) (tibicos)

Sweetener (not required if coconut water is used): 14 cup sugar (cane, brown, or maple syrup)

Optional: sliced ginger root or chopped or sliced fruit of your choosing

Optional: a pinch of salt Procedure: Before using, carefully clean all equipment.

Fill the container halfway with water, then gently mix in the kefir grains.

sweetener.

Optional: Add a pinch of sea salt to help the fermentation process along by adding trace minerals.

Place the jar in a dark, out-of-the-way location away from direct sunshine. Cheesecloth, towel, or a sprouting lid may be used to cover it loosely (which provides air circulation).

After 12 hours, and again after 24 hours, check your water kefir. In the jar, swish it around a little and then taste it with a clean spoon. Give it another 12 hours if it isn't sour enough for you. Fermentation will be quicker in hot temperatures and slower in cold weather. If you want to fine-tune your kefir, place the whole jar in the refrigerator, where it will ferment more slowly.

When you're ready to end the fermentation, filter the kefir grains out of the beverage using the strainer over a bowl. If you used fruit or ginger, you'll need to pick out the kefir grains using wooden/bamboo chopsticks; my preferred tool for this is a pair of chopsticks. Your kefir may be consumed right once or kept in the refrigerator in a jar or plastic container.

Use your kefir grains right away in a fresh batch of sugar water, or keep them in the refrigerator for up to two weeks (sitting in some sugar water).

Verifying Proper Fermentation

If your kombucha is fermenting correctly, you should be able to tell by the smell and the little bubbles. However, if you think anything has gone wrong and the culture has failed, you should investigate more. pH test strips are the most effective technique of inquiry. If the pH of your solution is not in the 2.5–3.0 range after 3–4 days of fermentation, it is not acidic enough and something is wrong. Remove everything, sanitise everything, and start again with a fresh culture. Also, if the kombucha has a strong kerosene scent rather than a yeast or vinegar smell, it indicates something else has gotten in there and you should discard it.

Fizzy Kombucha

If your kombucha is not as effervescent as you would like, you can conduct a secondary fermentation in a bottle. To fuel this second stage, you can use juice (which provides a nice flavour), or else use some more sweet tea. Either way, you will end up with a kombucha soda. Take a plastic bottle with a tight-fitting lid, such as a soda or water bottle. (You can use a glass jar or bottle also, but it is easiest to check the air pressure in a plastic vessel.) Fill it three-quarters of the way with your fermented kombucha and top this off with some additional juice. Tighten the lid and leave this at room temperature to continue fermenting. It probably will be ready in 2–7 days, but check it every day or so.

If you used a plastic bottle, then checking it is as simple as squeezing the sides of the bottle. If it has really puffed out so that squeezing is difficult, your drink should be ready. Open with caution, since the contents may be under pressure. Unless you've shaken the bottle, it really should not explode on you, but there will be a release of air pressure as there is when opening any soda bottle. Taste and decide if it's fizzy enough for you. If not, tighten the lid and give it another 12 hours or so.

Storing and Reusing Your Kombucha SCOBY

Storing a kombucha SCOBY is easier than storing kefir grains, simply because it takes longer to ferment a batch. This means that you can start fermenting some sweet tea with a kombucha SCOBY and just leave it for as long as a couple of weeks. The fermented liquid may be too acidic to drink, but your culture should still be alive after that time and you can begin using it again. While you can store your SCOBY in the refrigerator, this can cause the yeasts to go dormant, so the above method is better.

Rejuvelac

Rejuvelac is a fermented beverage made from sprouted cereal grains, such as wheat, barley, rye, oats, triticale, millet, amaranth, quinoa, brown rice, wild rice, or buckwheat. People have been making fermented drinks with grains for thousands of years, but the raw food advocate Ann Wigmore is credited with popularising rejuvelac as part of a holistic health diet. It's pretty sour and definitely qualifies as an acquired taste unless you add some sugar, honey, or other sweetener. Alternatively, this makes a great base ingredient for sodas, or you can mix it with juice, and it can be used to culture anything else in this book.

½ cup organic grains such as wheat, rye, barley, or oats (whole-seeded, not ground or cracked) (whole-seeded, not ground or cracked)

Water\sOptional: 1 tbsp yoghurt whey or water kefir

Rinse the grains. Put them in the jar or container and cover them with water. Let them soak overnight. In the morning, drain the water from the grains, rinse them, and put them back in the jar. The rinsing prevents mould. Continue to rinse twice per day for 1–2 days, until grains form small white tails, indicating that they have sprouted. Rinse them once more and put grains in the large container. You could use the same jar if it's big enough (be sure to rinse before reusing) (be sure to rinse before reusing). Cover the grains with one quart of water. Add yoghurt whey or other culture, if you choose to use this (if not, the natural yeasts and bacteria on grains will ferment the water) (if not, the natural yeasts and bacteria on grains will ferment the water). Cover the container loosely, checking it by tasting every 24 hours. This fermentation normally takes 1–3 days, and the later you let it go, the more sour it will be. Then pour out the liquid, which is the consumable part. The grains have left the better part of their nutrition in the liquid and are spent, so you can compost them. Feel free to add some sweetener or combine the rejuvelac with juice to make it drinkable.

This section is reserved for three special drinks. They could be considered sodas or smoothies, but all three are made a bit differently from the other drinks.

Probiotic Lemonade Makes about 2 quarts

This only takes a few more minutes than dissolving one of those chemical- filled lemonade envelopes in water. This drink is probiotic from the start by virtue of the cultured drink (kombucha, cider, etc.) you have added. But if you can wait for a richer ferment, prepare the drink in advance and let all the ingredients stand together for 24–48 hours. Also, see the separate Lemon-Lime Soda recipe, which is similar. Try this lemonade on your kids!

Juice of 5 lemons

½ cup kombucha, cider, water kefir, or yoghurt whey

1½–2 quarts water

¼–½ cup sugar or honey

Mix together all ingredients and let the drink sit in a jar or container for 24– 48 hours or until it reaches desired sourness. If it's too sour, feel free to thin it out with more water or add extra honey or sugar. Garnish with a sprig of mint or slices of lemon.

Watermelon Kombucha Cooler Makes about 2 cups

1 cup ripe watermelon

1½ cups kombucha or water kefir

Honey or sugar, to taste

Blend watermelon to purée it. If chunks remain, strain them out. For a frozen drink, freeze watermelon or purée first, then blend with kombucha or water kefir. If you do not freeze the purée, then you can stir it directly into the kombucha.

Pineapple Tapache Makes 3–4 quarts

This delicious beverage from Mexico may well be my favourite drink in this book. The recipe involves fermenting a whole pineapple (cut into chunks) in sweetened water with spices. You can culture it with water kefir grains (tibicos), yoghurt whey, or cider. Otherwise, just let the naturally present bacteria culture it themselves. Traditionally, people cut up the peel and put this in to get plenty of bacteria. If you use the rind, then please cut off the bottom and discard this part, as ripe pineapples often have a little mould at the base of the core.

3–4 quarts water

1 fresh pineapple, peeled and cut into chunks

3 cups natural cane sugar or brown sugar

1 tsp vanilla extract

1 cinnamon stick or one tsp ground cinnamon

Optional: 1 tbsp apple pie spice

Put the pineapple chunks in a very large container or jar, covering it with water. Use enough water to cover the pineapple—probably about half (2 quarts) of your water. Also add the sugar and spices. Then add your kefir/yogurt/cider culture, if you use any. Cover loosely and let it ferment. After 48 hours, add another quart of water and cover it loosely again. Let it sit for 12 hours this time before tasting. If it is sour enough for you, then drink some and refrigerate the rest. If it needs more time, add more water and give it an additional 12 hours to ferment. It should be ready at that point, and if it is too sour, you can add a little sugar, honey, or apple juice. You can eat the pineapple chunks or compost them. I feed some to my backyard chickens (the subject of another book) who love pineapple.

They need their probiotics, too!

Healthy Energy Drink

Now, let's cover energy drinks. In theory, these are a great idea, but in practise, most commercially produced energy drinks do not provide healthy results. They are designed to give you a short-term fix with massive quantities of caffeine and sugar, combined with a questionable cocktail of herbs, vitamins, and amino acids such as guanine and taurine. Guanine is a stimulant derived from the guarana plant, which is high in caffeine, while the amino acid taurine serves to concentrate caffeine in the body.

Energy drinks have been blamed, rightly or wrongly, for a number of deaths. Many experts consider them to be unhealthy and perhaps dangerous to consume, particularly in combination with other active substances such as alcohol, tobacco, and more caffeine. Instead of consuming substances that squeeze the body for a short-term energy rush, why not make your own probiotic energy drink using safe and wholesome foods? These drinks can nourish the body and boost energy levels naturally. You can find many of the ingredients you need in your kitchen or cupboard.

Start with a base of kefir, water kefir, rejuvelac, or kombucha. Then add any of the ingredients below, each of which has been proven to have a positive effect on a person's energy. As always, if you are suffering from a particular medical condition, consult a qualified physician or natural health expert before making your own energy drinks or consuming any of the following substances that your body may not have encountered before (such as ginseng) (such as ginseng).

Cinnamon and Honey: Cinnamon has a warming flavour that adds a special touch to many foods and drinks. Honey, especially raw and unpasteurized honey with its enzymes intact, delivers a simple carbohydrate boost to your body. In a recent study, researchers found that cinnamon enhanced participants' brain functions and cognitive processing. Participants who smelled cinnamon or chewed cinnamon gum achieved better scores on a computer test of several different cognitive and memory functions. Separate research showed that taking half a teaspoon of honey sprinkled with cinnamon, around 3:00 p.m.

each day, increases the body's vitality within a week at this time of the day when many people's body clocks are on a low ebb. It seems that a sprinkle of cinnamon is all you need to add to a homemade energy drink to get these benefits (and even the smell alone might do the job!). Large quantities of cinnamon can be toxic.

Citrus: Have you ever drank a glass of orange juice and felt more alert? When I stopped drinking coffee regularly many years ago, I often drank orange juice in the morning, and I swore it helped me wake up. It turns out I was not imagining this. Research has shown that both the smell of citrus and the acidity of the juice can awaken your body. Plus, it provides a great flavouring for any

kefir, kombucha, natural soda, or energy drink. Try squeezing a little orange, lemon, lime, mandarin, or grapefruit juice into your drink.

Green Tea: Green tea can help increase your energy levels in several ways. First, since it contains some caffeine, you get a short-term boost. Typically, green tea contains much less caffeine than a cup of coffee, an energy drink, or a caffeinated soda. If you want the other benefits of green tea without the caffeine, you can opt for naturally decaffeinated green tea. To put green tea's caffeine level in perspective, consider the following list of the typical quantities of caffeine in these common sources. I think you'll find that green tea contains a smaller amount of caffeine than most alternatives: • Green tea (8 oz): 25–40 mg of caffeine

Black tea (8 oz): 15–60 mg

Coca-Cola® (8 oz): 20–30 mg

Monster™/Red Bull™/Rockstar™ Energy Drinks (8.0–8.4 oz): 80–92 mg

5-Hour Energy™ (2 oz): 207 mg

Dark Chocolate (1.5 oz): 26 mg

Milk chocolate (1.5 oz): 9 mg

The second way that green tea boosts your energy level is with a natural substance it contains called L-theanine, which has been shown to increase alertness without the jitters of caffeine. And third, EGCG is a powerful antioxidant in green tea that scrubs your body of free radicals.

This should help you feel more energetic over time.

Ginseng: Thousands of years' worth of testing on humans has demonstrated ginseng's near-magical properties to the people of China, Korea, Japan, and beyond. More recently, Western studies have verified that panax ginseng (the most effective kind) really does boost energy. It may reach this result by improving blood flow to the brain. This is a natural increase that can be sustainable; it has none of the ups and downs associated with caffeine. Ginseng also is revered in Asia for its effect on sexual potency, which may also be related to the improved blood flow to the brain. Studies have proven that people who take ginseng before a test have better memory recognition and higher scores.

There are several kinds of ginseng, including American and Siberian, but panax ginseng (also known as red ginseng, Chinese red ginseng, or Korean ginseng) is the one that works best. I've tried a lot of herbs that are said to be good for one thing or another. Not one of them has ever worked on me the way panax ginseng does. If your energy is at a low ebb or you are feeling like you are getting a cold, drinking a strong cup of red ginseng tea might give you new life. It lifts me up a couple of levels on the energy metre and puts me back in a place where I feel like my body has the strength to fight off a pesky cold. If I felt like

taking a nap before consuming ginseng, I often feel like running a mile or two after taking it (not always right away but within a few hours) (not always right away but within a few hours).

What about its potency? I'll let you test it out for yourself. Of course, if you have a medical problem or are on medication, check with your doctor first, particularly because ginseng is the most powerful energy supplement in this chapter. Ginseng tea, extract, and powder are the most common methods to include it into a probiotic beverage. It seems to be most effective at dosages over 200 mg, although this information may or may not be included on the label of the tea or extract you get. Following the instructions on the label is the best place to start, and you may modify the quantities as needed. If you can't locate ginseng in your local Asian market or health food shop, try searching for "red ginseng" online. It's well worth the money.

Mint: Mint's aroma and flavour may refresh the senses. Use a sprig of mint as an edible garnish, or crush some mint leaves and soak them in water to create a mint extract to flavour beverages. Another easy alternative is to make peppermint, spearmint, or pennyroyal tea, let it cool, and then add it to beverages.

Putting Everything Together

A recipe for a homemade probiotic energy drink using all of these recommended boosters may be found below. You don't have to utilise all of them; simply the ones you like and have on hand would suffice. If you really need a boost, though, I recommend ginseng, which has a greater impact on energy levels than any other meal. You may already have some of the others in your kitchen or pantry, ranging from citrus to cinnamon to mint tea.

Time-Saving Tea Bags

If you don't have the time to make your own beverage, here's a quick fix that just costs a few bucks. Several tea firms, including Lipton®, Celestial SeasoningsTM, and Bigelow®/AriZona Iced Tea®, manufacture and sell tea bags with a variety of energy-boosting compounds. All of these items may be found at herbal tea shops or on the internet. Lemon ginseng green tea is made by Lipton, honey lemon ginseng green tea is made by Celestial Seasonings, and green tea with ginseng and honey is made by Bigelow (branded as AriZona). Rather of locating and measuring all of the components, you might spend a few dollars on a package of twenty-five tea bags. You could boil a half cup or so of water, steep the tea bag in it till it cools a little, then fill up the cup with water kefir, rejuvelac, or kombucha whenever you wanted an energy drink. If desired, add a bit extra honey, cinnamon, mint, or a splash of citrus. Wow, it was a breeze!

The recipes for the green drink (which comes first) and the energy drink are below (at the end of this chapter).

Makes 4–6 cups of spinach shake

The two cups of young spinach in this smoothie are hidden by sweet and dark fruit. Baby kale or other greens may also be used. Fresh or frozen fruit may be used in any recipe.

1 banana, ripe

12 CUP OLIVE JUICE

1 pound of blueberries

1 pineapple cup

1 quart of yoghurt

2 cups spinach (baby)

To taste, honey or sugar

In a blender, combine all of the ingredients. Blend, taste, and adjust with more honey or sugar as needed before serving.

2–3 cups of green chocolate chia

Chia seeds, which are extremely healthy and widely accessible at health food shops, are used in this dish. You could use poppy seeds, hemp seed hearts, flax seeds, or ground flaxseed meal instead of the seeds... or leave them altogether if you just want the green chocolate! If you're using chia seeds, soak them for 5 minutes in a small cup with a bit of the liquid you'll be using in the recipe (such as kombucha or kefir). Scrape in as many of the sticky seeds as you can before pouring it into your mixer. You may use as much spirulina, green powder, or spinach as you want.

1 cup chocolate ice cream (or 1 cup yoghurt + 1 packet cocoa mix)

chia seeds, 1–3 tbsp (presoaked as described above)

1–3 tablespoons (or more) 1 cup baby spinach leaves or spirulina or green juice powder

a quarter teaspoon of vanilla extract

1 cup rejuvelac, kombucha, or kefir

a handful of fresh mint leaves, if desired

Serve with a sprig of fresh mint as a garnish.

In a blender, combine all of the ingredients. Blend, taste, and adjust with more honey or sugar as needed before serving.

Smoothie with Kale, Banana, and Pear Approximately 2–3 cups

This dish mixes some nutritious vegetables with an abundance of delicious, custardy fruit (bananas and pears). Kale is a simple vegetable to cultivate in the home garden and is very cold-hardy; we can grow it nearly all year. If only harder, mature kale leaves are available, pull off the leafy portions and discard the stems. Another option is to juice your kale first and then add the juice to the smoothie. You may also use baby spinach leaves instead.

bananas (two)

1 cup milk (or CRASH substitute)

2 peeled and sliced ripe pears

2 quarts baby spinach or baby kale

12 cup cottage cheese or yoghurt

In a blender, combine all of the ingredients. Blend, taste, and adjust with more honey or sugar as needed before serving.

Kvass made with beets and greens yields 4–5 cups

Kvass is a traditional Russian beverage prepared mostly from beets or dry rye bread. It's a sour-salty drink. This dish uses just beets, greens, and celery instead of rye bread. It should be mixed because of the extra veggies. You may use yoghurt whey, sauerkraut or natural pickle juice, or vegetable starting culture, or you can omit the starter and depend on naturally existing lactobacteria to ferment the veggies more slowly (organic beets and celery have plenty of naturally present cultures). Kvass, like many fermented foods and beverages, takes some getting used to. Those who like it often extol its health advantages, with some even drinking kvass on a regular basis.

3 big peeled and cut into cubes beets

1 gallon of water

1 celery stalk, chopped

a small handful of baby spinach or greens

2 tsp starting culture/whey

Optional: 12–2 teaspoons salt

Optional: 2 tbsp ginger (chopped) or 1 garlic clove (crushed)

Place all of the ingredients in a blender and mix until smooth.

Transfer the drink to a container or jar. Allow your beverage to

ferment for 3–5 days at room temperature, covered loosely. If

desired, season with salt or sugar before drinking.

Smoothie with Savory Veggies

This might be named V7, V9, or whatever number of vegetables

you add, but I don't want to confuse it with a canned vegetable

juice. By adding salt and jalapeño pepper, you may make it as salty

or spicy as you want. If you have some, add some sauerkraut or

natural pickles for an additional probiotic boost! If this smoothie is

too fibrous for you, another alternative is to puree these vegetables

and then combine the liquid with the other ingredients in the

blender.

1 quart of tomato juice

a quarter-cup of carrot juice

12 cup kombucha, rejuvelac, or water kefir

12 cucumber slices, peeled

1 celery stem, tiny

a quarter-cup of bell pepper

12 cup baby spinach or kale greens (baby spinach or kale greens)

1 smashed garlic clove or a tiny handful of fresh chives

1 teaspoon lime or lemon juice

To taste, season with salt, black pepper, and cayenne pepper.

12 jalapeno pepper (optional)

14 cup sauerkraut or natural pickles (optional)

In a blender, combine all of the ingredients. Blend, taste, and adjust with more honey or sugar as needed before serving.

Green Smoothie with Carrots and Seaweed Approximately 2 cups

Dried seaweed may be found at Asian and health food shops.

While kelp (kombu) is preferred, most other types will suffice. To produce a varied variety of nutrients and flavour, try adding a few different types of seaweed. Soak the seaweed for at least 2 hours or until it is soft to rehydrate it. The seaweed will be firm yet wet all the way through.

12 cup seaweed (dry) (soaked in water for at least 2 hours or until tender)

12 cup carrot juice 1–112 cup carrot juice

12 cup kombucha, rejuvelac, or water kefir

14 inch peeled and sliced fresh ginger

Optional: 1 banana if you want it to be a little sweeter. Energy Drinks That Are Good For You

Approximately 2 cups

1 cup boiling water

1 panax ginseng tea bag (100–500 mg strength) or 200 milligrammes panax ginseng (extract or powder)

1 green tea bag or 1 teaspoon dried green tea leaves

Lemon, lime, grapefruit, or orange juice

1 cup kombucha, kefir, or apple cider

To taste, honey or sugar

Pour water over the ginseng and green tea (at a temperature just below boiling). Allow 3 minutes for steeping. Remove the tea bags or pour the tea liquid into a separate cup or container, straining the tea leaves if necessary. Allow the tea to cool or put it in the refrigerator until it reaches a temperature of less than 100°F. If desired, add honey or sugar. Then mix in the rest of the ingredients. Serve with a sprig of mint or a piece of citrus as a garnish.

Energy Drink with Grapefruit and Mint Approximately 2–3 cups

2 cups water kefir or kombucha

14 cup Mint Soda Syrup 1 grapefruit juice

Serve by combining all of the ingredients. Serve with fresh mint as a garnish.

Energy Drink with Mandarin Orange Spice

2 quarts apple cider

3–4 mandarin oranges or tangerines, juice

Cinnamon, pinch

a thin piece of peeled ginger or a sprinkle of ginger powder

Optional: 1 clove or a pinch of spices

Combine the orange juice and spices in a small bowl, and chill for

a few minutes or hours if you have time. Then mix in the cider.

4 Carrot Gold, 4 Carrot Gold, 4 Carrot Gold, 4 Carrot Gold, 4 Antioxidant Rush, Antioxidant Rush, Antioxidant Rush, Antioxidant Rush, Anti Apple Cinnamon Kombucha, 156 oz. Apple Glory, 262 Apple Green, 69 Smoothie with Apples and Melon, 78 Apple Pie Smoothie (139 calories), Apple Sprouts, 80 oz. Smoothie with Apricots and Melon (89), 76 Asian Green Smoothie, 66 Kombucha Basics 251 Beet the Blues, Beet the Blues, Beet the Blues, Beet the 221 Kvass with Beets and Greens, 298 Dandelion Beet-er, Beetle Juice (225 mL), Green Smoothie with Berries and Melon, 199 Berry Melon Heaven, No. 102 Berry Rocket Green Smoothie, 152 calories Blackberry Sage Kombucha, 106 oz. 265 Oh my goodness, Mary! Smoothie #215, Blue Banana Green Green Smoothie with 99 Breakfast Fillers, Broccoli, 120 Broccoli, 120 Broccoli, 120 Broccoli, 120 Bro Cacao Dessert Smoothie (179 calories), Cacao Green Smoothie (#69), Green Smoothie with 101 Carrots and Seaweed, 301 Chard Candy, 301 Chard Candy, 301 Chard Candy, 135 Choco Passion Green Smoothie, 135 Choco Passion Green Smoothie, 135

Choco Passion Green Smooth 113 Apple Cinnamon Smoothie Smoothie with Coco and Mango, 146 Cocoa Mo, 140 Col. Mustard Greens, 137 Cold Killah, 85 217 Winter Healer Complete, Cool Slaw, 165 192 Cosmo Chiller, 192 Cosmo Chiller, 192 Cosmo Chiller, Lagoon, 97 Crystal Clean, Green Smoothie, Green Smoothie, Green Smoothie, Green Smoothie, Green Smoothie,

Dande-Lemon, 203 Dapper Dan, 182 Emerald Deluxe, 183 Emerald Fantasy, 203 Dapper Dan, 182 Emerald Deluxe, 183 Emerald Fantasy, 203 Dapper Dan, 18 188 Excitement Juice in Your Mouth, Feast of a Champion, 172 173 Fig Kombucha, 173 Fig Kombucha, 173 Fig Kombucha 272 Fizzy Kombucha, Fizzy Kombucha, Fizzy Kombucha, Fizzy Kom 281 Forever Young, 229 Fresh!, 281 Forever Young, 229 Fresh!, 281 Forever Young, 2 71 Monkey Juice, Frothy 186 Fruity Power Green Smoothie, 119 Garden Smoothie, 186 Fruity Power Green Smoothie, 186 Fruity Power Green Smoothie, 186 Fruity 71\sGazpacho, 95 Ginger Green Smoothie, 82 Ginger Snap, 95 Ginger

Green Smoothie, 95 Ginger Green Smoothie, 95 Ginger Green Smoothi 213 Gold 'n' Delicious, 213 Gold 'n' Delicious, 213 Gold 'n' Grandma Love, 219 Grapefruit Mint Energy Drink (64 oz.) Grapefruit and Pineapple Diet Yogurt Smoothie, 303 calories Green Broccoli Smoothie (143), 77 Chia Green Chocolate, 296 Smoothie de Noel Verde Verde Verde Verde Verde Verde Verde Green Clean, 81 211 Green Apricot Cream Smoothie, Green Explosion, No. 82 Green Goddess, 184 80 Green King, 186 Green Grape Smoothie Green Kiwi Smoothie 207, Green Lcuma Smoothie 76, Green Orange Smoothie 72 Green Passion, 75 Smoothie with 77 Green Pears, Green Smoothie with Chaga Tea, 70 calories 74 Energy Drinks That Are Good For You, 302 Highly Potent Pallooza (Highly Potent Pallooza) 170 Hot Rocket, 201 Hot Mamma Green Juice

Smoothie with Iron, 75 grammes of jasmine kombucha 266 Smoothie with Kale, Banana, and Pear 297 Kombucha Kombucha Kombucha Kombucha Kombucha Kombuch Lemon Ginger Kombucha, 280 mL

231 Lola Dreaming, 260 Lettuce Sleep Lunchtime Booster Green Smoothie, 152 calories 121 Mandarin Orange Spice Energy Drink, 121 Mandarin Orange Spice Energy Drink, 121 Mandarin Orange Spice Energy Drink 305 Mangomole, Mangomole, Mangomole, Mangomole Smoothie with Melon, Berry, and Yogurt, 93 Melon Refresher, 142 Multi Nutri Juice, 159 164 Orange Ecstasy, Orange Ecstasy, Orange Ecstasy, Orange Ecsta Smoothie with 155 Orange and Go Green, Smoothie with Papaya and Lime, 111 81 Warrior of Peace, 171 Peach Punch, 171 Peach Punch, 171 Peach Punch, 17 Green Smoothie with 123 Pears, Pear Delight, 107 Perfect Purifier, 157 162 PERFECTLY SIMPLE EXPRESSION, 189 Pia Kale-ada, Pia Kale-ada, Pia Kale-ada, Pia Pineapple Detox Green Smoothie (131 Pineapple Detox Green Smoothie), Pineapple Kombucha, 103 268 Pineapple Tapache, 268 Pineapple Tapache, 268 Pineapple Tapache 285 Pink Magic Woman, 285 Pink Magic Woman, 285 Pink Magic Woman, 2 Pink Silk, 223 155\sPlumkin, Pomegranate Kombucha (125 g) (Kombucha and Juice), Pomegranate Pow Wow, 258 Smoothie with Pomegranate

and Strawberries, 154 144 Pomegreen Smoothie, 144 Pomegreen Smoothie, 144 Pomegreen Smoothi Lemonade with 78 probiotics, 284 Flu Fighter, Quick and Dirty 109 Quick Orange Breakfast Green Smoothie, 150 Quick Green Smoothie Radish, Radish, Radish, Radish, Radish, Radish, Radish, 270 Raspberry Mint Kombucha, 177 Raspberry Mint Kombucha

Heavenly Concoction of Red and Green, Red Queen, 169 197 Refresh, 68 Rejuvelac, 197 Refresh, 68 Rejuvelac, 197 Refresh, 68 Rocket Fuel, 282 Ruby Rapture, 209 Sangria Blanca, 156 91 Vegetables Must Be Saved Smoothie with Savory Veggies, 227 Sea-buckthorn Smoothie (300 mL), 74 Spinach Shake Recipes, 295 sassy and sexy surprise Shanti Om Elixir, 190 Simply Sweet, 185 Smooth Sensation, 127 Sprout Smoothie, 187 Green Smoothie with Strawberry & Melon Delight, 68 115 Strawberrylicious, Strawberrylicious, Strawberrylicious, Strawberrylicious, Strawberry 72 Paradise Sunrise, There are 154 Super Detoxes to choose from. 167 Smoothie de

Verdure Verdure Verdure Verdure Verdure Verd Sweet Mint, 114 Sweet Pear Sensation, 129 Smoothie with Sweet Yogurt and Watermelon, 153 145 Sweet and Tart Cooler, Tropical Green Smoothie, No. 151 Tropical Punch, 116 Tummy Rub, 157 193 Pineapple-Kale Blast (Ultimate Pineapple-Kale Blast), Unbelievably Creamy Lush Dream, 180 oz. Very Berry, 189 161\sVeggie-All, Vitamin C Minty Rush, 205 181 Morning Cocktail (Wake Me Up), 153 Green Smoothie (Wake Up), Water Kefir (118 g) (or Coconut Water Kefir), Watermelon Kombucha Cooler (#278) 285\sWhat-A-Lemon, 175 Whole Enchilada, 87 Whole Enchilada

Zingy Spring Green Smoothie, 104 Wild Honey, 133 Yellow Sunset, 191 Zen Dragonfly, 187 Zingy Spring Green Smoothie

CPSIA information can be obtained
at www.ICGtesting.com
Printed in the USA
LVHW021322171121
703571LV00008B/383

9 781803 796079